Get Through

MCEM Part A: MCQs

Get Through
MCEM Part A: MCQs

Iain Beardsell MB ChB FCEM
Consultant in Emergency Medicine, Southampton University Hospital Trust

Simon Bell BSc MBBS MRCP FCEM
Consultant in Emergency Medicine, Poole NHS Foundation Trust

Sarah Robinson BM MRCS(A&E) Ed FCEM
Consultant in Emergency Medicine, Southampton University Hospital Trust;
Alison Gourdie Medal for outstanding performance in FCEM

Helen Rumbold BA MBBS MA MCEM
Specialist Trainee in Emergency Medicine, Wessex Deanery

Consulting Editor

Diana Hulbert BSc MBBS FRCS FCEM
Consultant in Emergency Medicine, Southampton University Hospital Trust;
Immediate Past President of the Royal Society of Medicine's Emergency Medicine Section

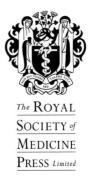

The ROYAL
SOCIETY *of*
MEDICINE
PRESS *Limited*

© 2009 Royal Society of Medicine Press Ltd

Published by the Royal Society of Medicine Press Ltd
1 Wimpole Street, London W1G 0AE, UK
Tel: +44 (0)20 7290 2921
Fax: +44 (0)20 7290 2929
Email: publishing@rsm.ac.uk
Website: www.rsmpress.co.uk

British Library Cataloguing in Publication Data
A catalogue record for this book is available from the British Library

ISBN: 978-1-85315-804-9

Distribution in Europe and Rest of World:
Marston Book Services Ltd
PO Box 269
Abingdon
Oxon OX14 4YN, UK
Tel: +44 (0)1235 465500
Fax: +44 (0)1235 465555
Email: direct.order@marston.co.uk

Distribution in the USA and Canada:
Royal Society of Medicine Press Ltd
c/o BookMasters Inc
30 Amberwood Parkway
Ashland, OH 44805, USA
Tel: +1 800 247 6553/+1 800 266 5564
Fax: +1 419 281 6883
Email: order@bookmasters.com

Distribution in Australia and New Zealand:
Elsevier Australia
30-52 Smidmore Street
Marrickville, NSW 2204, Australia
Tel: +61 2 9517 8999
Fax: +61 2 9517 2249
Email: service@elsevier.com.au

Typeset by Techset Composition Limited, Salisbury, UK
Printed and bound in Great Britain by Bell & Bain, Glasgow

Contents

Foreword I

It is an absolute pleasure to welcome this book to the resources available for trainees in emergency medicine preparing for the membership exam. This is a tough exam and it is a great credit to the commitment, and enthusiasm of trainees who dedicate themselves to preparing for and subsequently passing the exam. In turn, this provides the specialty of emergency medicine with an outstanding group of trainees who will take their skills and talents into the emergency medicine training programme to eventually emerge as exactly the highly skilled and experienced consultants needed to deliver an emergency medicine service of the highest quality and calibre. This is obviously a fundamental expectation of the public and the patients who put great trust and confidence in the quality of care provided in our emergency departments.

The authors should be congratulated for their diligence and hard work in compiling this book which will now become an essential companion for trainees preparing for the membership exam.

John Heyworth
President, College of Emergency Medicine

Foreword II

The passing of the Membership of the College of Emergency Medicine (MCEM) Part A exam is a significant achievement and anything that can help future candidates is most welcome.

This book bridges a significant gap in training materials. By providing questions around the basic sciences within an emergency medicine context wherever possible, the authors, all practising emergency medicine physicians, have successfully covered large and important areas of the basic sciences curriculum. The provision of brief, but informative, explanations greatly enhances the book and makes for effective revision. I am sure that future candidates will avidly absorb its contents. I congratulate the authors on a job well done.

Mike Clancy
Dean, College of Emergency Medicine

Preface

Passing the MCEM Part A represents the first step on the postgraduate exam ladder to achieving specialist accreditation in emergency medicine. Unless trainee emergency doctors successfully pass this exam they are unable to progress to further years of specialist training. Testing candidates in material that was previously covered perhaps only in the early years of medical school, success in this exam, for many, has proved difficult to achieve.

The MCEM Part A is a new exam; the first candidates to sit the MFAEM in 2003 (before the Faculty of Emergency Medicine became the College of Emergency Medicine) were not offered the choice of a multiple-choice paper specifically aimed at emergency doctors, but instead had to sit the primary paper of another specialty. The development of this exam is one of the more obvious steps forward in the evolution of emergency medicine and the training of emergency doctors in recent years.

With such a new exam there is an inevitable lack of published material to aid candidates in their preparation. This book aims to fill that gap. Written by practising emergency physicians, in a format mirroring that of the MCEM exam, it covers all areas of the syllabus. Accompanying each answer is a brief, but comprehensive, text explanation to augment revision. As such this book should prove useful from the moment that you decide to sit the exam to last minute cramming the night before.

We believe that emergency medicine is the most rewarding hospital specialty, with a breadth and diversity not encountered in any other, and we wish you luck in your future careers. We hope that this book will aid you in realising your ambition to become specialist emergency physicians.

IB, SB, SR, HR, DH

Exam advice from the College of Emergency Medicine

History of the MCEM exam

The first sitting of the MCEM exam was in 2003 when there were 30 candidates. Since then there has been a lot of work on exam question and curriculum development. In December 2008 the exam was taken by 353 candidates in the UK, 12 in India and 19 in Singapore.

The basic science curriculum content has been determined by front-line emergency doctors (working over a 4-year period using Delphi methodology) as directly relevant to practice in emergency medicine. The exam is focused on the basic sciences relevant to the practice of emergency medicine. The curriculum is available on the College of Emergency Medicine website (www.collemergencymed.ac.uk/cem).

The MCEM Part A exam tests the basic science knowledge needed by emergency doctors and must be passed if the trainee is to progress beyond ST3. Basic sciences also feature in both the MCEM Part B and C, and the FCEM exams.

Question format

The MCEM A exam is conducted twice yearly and is an MCQ paper consisting of 50 questions derived from the curriculum, with four parts to each (i.e. a total of 200 questions per paper). The questions are true/false. There is no negative marking. The exam is of 2 hours' duration.

The question distribution across subjects is as follows:

Anatomy	10 questions (20%)
Physiology	10 questions (20%)
Pharmacology	5 questions (10%)
Microbiology	5 questions (10%)
Clinical	5 questions (10%)
Biochemistry	5 questions (10%)
Haematology	5 questions (10%)
Pathology	3 questions (6%)
Statistics	2 questions (4%)

Tips on revising for MCEM Part A

Many candidates do not understand the size of the task involved and are consequently ill prepared. Trainees need to appreciate that this exam represents a substantial undertaking, typically requiring 9 months' revision time (or the order of 1000 hours). This figure is less if the applicant has a good grounding in undergraduate basic sciences or has a basic science degree. In contrast, graduates from some UK medical schools may be in the position of having to learn large amounts of anatomy and other basic sciences for the first time. In these cases proportionally greater time will be needed. Therefore potential candidates for this exam must look at the curriculum, discuss the exam with their trainer and, if they wish to take it, commit themselves (in the form of an educational agreement), ideally early in their F2 year, in order to give sufficient time for revision and two attempts at the exam. The trainers and the College of Emergency Medicine are resources that can help the candidate. However, it is the candidate's application and determination that are essential to success. The candidate will need to spend a significant amount of personal time reading and learning the recommended textbooks, as well as using electronic media.

Tips for learning in the workplace

1. Use patients as a trigger (e.g. radiographs, blood gases, hand injuries) for teaching some important basic science point. This requires putting a small amount of time to one side to learn a specific aspect of applied basic science per shift. This brings alive the basic sciences by demonstrating the relevance of the subject and also leads to a discussion on how these facts can be remembered at 02:00 while doing a night shift!
2. Consider developing the areas that you are covering in your revision by teaching the topic to your peers.
3. Set targets for coverage of the basic sciences and aim to review these with your trainer at least fortnightly.

Recommended reading

Anatomy

Ellis, H. *Clinical Anatomy*, 11th edn. Oxford: Wiley-Blackwell, 2006.
Moore KL, Dalley AF, Agur AMR. *Clinically Orientated Anatomy*, 6th edn. Baltimore, MD: Lippincott Williams & Wilkins, 2009.

Physiology

Ganong WF. *Review of Medical Physiology*, 22nd edn. New York: McGraw-Hill Medical, 2005.
McPhee SJ, Vishwanath RL, Ganong W. *Pathophysiology of Disease: An introduction to clinical medicine*, 5th edn. New York: McGraw-Hill Medical, 2006.

Pharmacology

British National Formulary. London: Pharmaceutical Press.
Neal M. *Medical Pharmacology at a Glance*, 6th edn. Oxford: Wiley-Blackwell, 2009.
Reid J, Rubin P, Whiting B. *Lecture Notes on Clinical Pharmacology*, 6th edn. Oxford: Wiley-Blackwell, 2001.

Microbiology

Champe P, Harvey R, Fisher B. *Microbiology*, 2nd edn. Baltimore, MD: Lippincott, Williams & Wilkins, 2006.

Clinical

Kumar P, Clark M. *Kumar and Clark's Clinical Medicine*, 6th edn. Philadelphia, PA: Saunders Ltd, 2005.
Wyatt J, Illingworth R, Graham C, Clancy M, Robertson C. *Oxford Handbook of Emergency Medicine*, 3rd edn. Oxford: Oxford University Press, 2006.

Biochemistry

Gaw A, Murphy MJ, Cowan RA et al. *Clinical Biochemistry: An illustrated colour text*, 4th edn. Edinburgh: Churchill Livingstone, 2008.

Haematology

Howard M, Hamilton P. *Haematology: An illustrated colour text*, 3rd edn. Edinburgh: Churchill Livingstone, 2007.

Pathology

Carton J, Daly R, Ramini P. *Clinical Pathology*. Oxford: Oxford University Press, 2006.

Statistics

Harris M, Taylor G. *Medical Statistics Made Easy*, 2nd edn. Oxford: Scion Publishing Ltd, 2008.

Abbreviations

5-HT	5-hydroxytryptamine or serotonin
βhCG	β human chorionic gonadotrophin
γGT	γ-glutamyl transpeptidase
ACE	angiotensin-converting enzyme
ACL	anterior cruciate ligament
ACTH	adrenocorticotrophin or adrenocorticotrophic hormone
ADH	antidiuretic hormone
AIDS	acquired immune deficiency syndrome
ALL	acute lymphoblastic leukaemia
ALP	alkaline phosphatase
ALT	alanine transaminase (or aminotransferase)
AML	acute myeloid leukaemia
ANA	anti-nuclear antibody
ANCA	anti-neutrophil cytoplasmic antibody
APLS	Advanced Paediatric Life Support
APTR	activated partial thromboplastin time ratio
aPTT	activated partial thromboplastin time
ARDS	acute respiratory distress syndrome
ARR	absolute risk reduction
AST	aspartate transaminase (or aminotransferase)
ATLS	Advanced Trauma Life Support
ATP	adenosine triphosphate
ATPase	adenosine triphosphatase
AV	atrioventricular
BCG	bacille Calmette–Guérin
BE	base excess
BNF	*British National Formulary*
BP	blood pressure
BSA	body surface area
CCK	cholecystokinin
CER	control event rate
CLL	chronic lymphocytic leukaemia
CMV	cytomegalovirus
CNS	central nervous system
CO	cardiac output
CPN	common peroneal nerve
CPR	cardiopulmonary resuscitation
CRH	corticotrophin-releasing hormone
CRP	C-reactive protein
CSF	cerebrospinal fluid
CT	computed tomography
CVA	cerebrovascular accident
D&V	diarrhoea and vomiting
DBP	diastolic blood pressure
DHEA	dihydroepiandrosterone
DIC	disseminated intravascular coagulation
DKA	diabetic ketoacidosis

2,3-DPG	2,3-diphosphogycerate
EBV	Epstein–Barr virus
ECF	extracellular fluid
ECG	electrocardiogram
ED	emergency department
EDV	end-diastolic volume
EER	experimental event rate
EOM	external oblique muscle
ESR	erythrocyte sedimentation rate
ESV	end-systolic volume
FEV_1	forced expiratory volume in 1 second
FFA	free fatty acid
FRC	functional residual capacity
FVC	forced vital capacity
G6PDH	glucose-6-phosphate dehydrogenase
GABA	γ-aminobutyric acid
GCS	Glasgow Coma Scale
GFR	glomerular filtration rate
GH	growth hormone
GHRH	growth hormone-releasing hormone
GI	gastrointestinal
GTN	glyceryl trinitrate
GUM	genitourinary medicine
Hb	haemoglobin
HbA	haemoglobin A
HbF	fetal haemoglobin
HbS	haemoglobin of sickle cell anaemia
HBsAg	hepatitis B surface antigen
Hib	*Haemophilus influenzae* type b
HIV	human immunodeficiency virus
HMG-CoA	hydroxymethylglutaryl coenzyme A
HR	heart rate
HRT	hormone replacement therapy
HSV	herpes simplex virus
HUS	haemolytic uraemic syndrome
HZV	herpes zoster virus
ICF	intracellular fluid
IGF	insulin-like growth factor
IL	interleukin
INR	international normalised ratio
IOM	internal oblique muscle
IT	intrathecal
IV	intravenous
IVC	inferior vena cava
KCCT	kaolin cephalin clotting time
LAD	left anterior descending artery
LCA	left coronary artery
LDH	lactate dehydrogenase
LDL	low-density lipoprotein
LR	likelihood ratio
MAP	mean arterial pressure

MCA	middle cerebral artery
MCV	mean corpuscular volume
MDR-TB	multi-drug-resistant tuberculosis
MMR	measles, mumps and rubella
NAC	N-acetylcysteine
NK	natural killer
NNH	number needed to harm
NNT	number needed to treat
NSAID	non-steroidal anti-inflammatory drug
PA	pernicious anaemia
PABA	p-aminobenzoic acid
PAS	periodic acid–Schiff
PCR	polymerase chain reaction
PE	pulmonary embolism
PEA	pulseless electrical activity
PEEP	positive end-expiratory pressure
PEP	post-exposure prophylaxis
PID	pelvic inflammatory disease
PNH	paroxysmal nocturnal haemoglobinuria
PP	pulse pressure
PPI	proton pump inhibitor
PT	prothrombin time
PTH	parathyroid hormone
PTT	partial thromboplastin time
PVN	paraventricular nucleus
RCA	right coronary artery
RF	rheumatoid factor
RSV	respiratory syncytial virus
SA	sinoatrial
SBP	systolic blood pressure
SCD	sickle cell disease
SIADH	syndrome of inappropriate antidiuretic hormone secretion
SIRS	systemic inflammatory response syndrome
SLE	systemic lupus erythematosus
SOB	shortness of breath
SON	hypothalamic supraoptic nucleus
SV	stroke volume
T_3	triiodothyronine
T_4	thyroxine
TAM	transverse abdominis muscle
TB	tuberculosis
TBG	thyroid (or thyroxine)-binding globulin
TBW	total body water
TCA	tricyclic antidepressant
TG	triglyceride
TIBC	total iron-binding capacity
TFT	thyroid function test
TIA	transient ischaemic attack
TMJ	temporomandibular junction
TNF	tumour necrosis factor

TRH	thyrotrophin-releasing hormone
TSH	thyroid-stimulating hormone
UTI	urinary tract infection
VF	ventricular fibrillation
$\dot{V}/\dot{Q}$	ventilation–perfusion ratio
VT	ventricular tachycardia
vWD	von Willebrand's disease
vWF	von Willebrand's factor
WPW	Wolff–Parkinson–White (syndrome)

I. Anatomy: Questions

1. **Pectoral region**
   a. Pectoralis major is innervated by the axillary nerve
   b. Trapezius is innervated by the accessory nerve
   c. Injury to the long thoracic nerve causes winging of the scapula
   d. Latissimus dorsi laterally rotates the humerus

2. **Rotator cuff**
   a. This is formed by supraspinatus, infraspinatus, subscapularis and teres major
   b. Infraspinatus externally rotates the arm
   c. Supraspinatus is supplied by the supraspinatus nerve
   d. Supraspinatus abducts the arm at the glenohumeral joint

3. **Brachial artery**
   a. This arises from the axillary artery
   b. It ends opposite the neck of the radius at the inferior border of the cubital fossa
   c. Its terminal branches are the radial and interosseous arteries
   d. It lies on the lateral aspect of the median nerve in the cubital fossa

4. **Posterior upper arm**
   a. This contains the triceps muscle which extends the forearm
   b. The triceps muscle is supplied by the radial nerve
   c. The radial nerve winds around the humerus in the spiral groove
   d. The lateral epicondyle of the humerus gives rise to the common origin of the tendon for the flexor muscles of the forearm

5. **Elbow joint**
   a. The trochlea articulates with the capitulum
   b. The lateral collateral ligament extends from the lateral epicondyle of the humerus to the radial tuberosity
   c. The medial collateral ligament extends from the medial epicondyle of the humerus to the olecranon and coronoid process of the ulna
   d. Avulsion of the medial epicondyle of the humerus may result in median nerve damage

6. **Blood supply of the forearm**
   a. The common interosseous artery arises from the ulnar artery
   b. The ulnar artery provides branches for the carpal and palmar arches
   c. The ulnar artery enters the hand deep to the flexor retinaculum
   d. The cephalic and basilic veins run on the lateral and medial aspects of the forearm respectively

7. **Injuries to the superior aspect of the brachial plexus**
   a. Often called Klumpke's palsy
   b. Result in paralysis of muscles supplied by C5 and C6 nerve roots
   c. The patient is unable to supinate the forearm
   d. The clinical appearance is of an abducted shoulder, medially rotated arm and extended elbow

8. **Wrist and hand injuries**
   a. Mallet finger occurs as a result of avulsion of the extensor tendon from the base of the dorsal aspect of the distal phalanx
   b. Scaphoid fractures are prone to avascular necrosis
   c. Distal radial fractures are associated with delayed rupture of extensor pollicis longus
   d. Ulnar nerve injury results in claw hand

9. **Anterior compartment of the thigh**
   a. This contains quadriceps femoris, pectineus, sartorius, iliopsoas and tensor fascia lata
   b. Pectineus, sartorius and quadriceps femoris are innervated by the femoral nerve
   c. Quadriceps femoris consists of four muscles
   d. The muscles of the anterior compartment flex the hip joint and extend the knee joint

10. **Femoral triangle**
    a. The three sides of the triangle are formed by the sartorius muscle, inguinal ligament and adductor magnus muscle
    b. The femoral artery and vein leave the femoral triangle at the inferior aspect and enter the adductor canal
    c. The long saphenous vein joins the femoral vein in the femoral triangle
    d. The floor of the femoral triangle is formed by the iliopsoas and pectineus muscles

11. **Sciatic nerve**
    a. This arises from L4 and L5, and S1–3
    b. It divides into the tibial and common fibular (peroneal) nerves
    c. It lies in the upper outer quadrant of the buttocks
    d. Is often damaged in anterior dislocation of the hip

12. **Popliteal fossa**
    a. The superior boundaries are formed by the long head of biceps femoris laterally and semitendinosus medially; the inferior border is formed by the lateral and medial head of gastrocnemius
    b. The sciatic nerve divides at the superior aspect of the popliteal fossa
    c. The common peroneal nerve passes along the superior medial aspect of the popliteal fossa
    d. The popliteal artery lies anterior to the popliteal vein

13. **Posterior compartment of the lower leg**
    a. This is supplied by the tibial nerve
    b. It is supplied by the posterior tibial artery
    c. The superficial compartment contains gastrocnemius, soleus and popliteus
    d. The deep compartment contains popliteus, flexor hallucis longus, flexor digitorum longus and tibialis posterior

14. **Anterior compartment of the lower leg**
    a. This is supplied by the anterior tibial nerve
    b. It contains tibialis anterior, extensor hallucis longus, extensor digitorum longus and peroneus tertius, which dorsiflex and invert the foot at the ankle joint
    c. It is supplied by the anterior tibial artery
    d. The patellar tendon inserts into the tibial tuberosity

15. **Lateral compartment of the lower leg**
    a. Peroneus brevis inserts into the base of the fifth metatarsal
    b. The lateral compartment of the lower leg is supplied by the deep peroneal nerve
    c. Peroneus longus inserts into the base of the first metatarsal
    d. The tendons of peroneus longus and brevis pass anterior to the lateral malleolus at the ankle joint

16. **Ankle joint**
    a. This is formed by the distal tibia, lateral malleolus of the fibula and talus
    b. The medial aspect is supported by the deltoid ligament
    c. The lateral ligament of the ankle joint has two components
    d. The ankle joint is more stable in plantar flexion than dorsiflexion

17. **Common peroneal nerve injury**
    a. This results in an inability to dorsiflex and invert the foot
    b. It can be caused by a poorly fitting below-knee plaster cast
    c. It leads to foot drop
    d. It results in a variable loss of sensation of the anterolateral aspect of the leg and dorsum of the foot

18. **Innervation of the foot**
    a. Most of the dorsum of the foot is innervated by the superficial peroneal nerve
    b. The sural nerve arises from the femoral nerve
    c. The saphenous nerve supplies some of the lateral aspect of the foot
    d. The tibial nerve gives rise to the medial and lateral plantar nerve

19. **Foot**
    a. The hindfoot consists of the calcaneum and talus
    b. The spring ligament runs from sustentaculum tali and inserts on the superior aspect of the navicular bone
    c. The lateral arch is formed by the calcaneous, cuboid and fourth and fifth metatarsals
    d. The medial arch is formed by the calcaneous, navicular and cuneiform bones, and first, second and third metatarsals

20. **First rib**
    a. The first rib articulates with the seventh cervical (C7) vertebra
    b. The first rib is easily fractured
    c. The subclavian vein crosses over the superior surface of the first rib anteriorly to scalenus anterior
    d. As the subclavian artery exits the superior mediastinum and enters the arm, it passes inferiorly to the first rib

21. **Diaphragm**
    a. It is innervated by the phrenic nerves which arise bilaterally from C2–4
    b. The aortic opening is at the level of T10
    c. The oesophageal opening is at the level of T12
    d. The inferior vena cava passes though the central tendon of the diaphragm

22. **Trachea**
    a. This arises at the level of the third cervical vertebra
    b. It divides into the two main bronchi at the level of the sternal angle (T4–5)
    c. The left main bronchus is wider and runs more vertically than the right main bronchus
    d. It is supported by circular rings of cartilage

23. **Pericardium**
    a. This consists of three layers: fibrous, serous parietal and serous visceral
    b. The function of the serous pericardial layers is to prevent overexpansion of the heart
    c. The pericardial cavity is between the fibrous and serous parietal layers of the pericardium
    d. The pericardium is supplied by the phrenic and vagus nerves and the sympathetic trunk

24. **Borders and surface anatomy of the heart**
    a. Right border = right atrium
    b. Inferior border = right ventricle and some of the left ventricle
    c. Left border = left ventricle and some of the left atrium
    d. Superior border = right and left atria, ascending aorta and pulmonary trunk, and superior vena cava

25. **Heart valve auscultation areas**
    a. Mitral area: fifth intercostal space, left midclavicular line
    b. Tricuspid area: fourth intercostal space, left sternal border
    c. Aortic area: left upper sternal border
    d. Pulmonary area: right upper sternal border

26. **Oesophagus**
    a. This arises at C4 and ends at T10
    b. It lies anterior to the left main bronchus
    c. It passes through the diaphragm anterior to the aorta
    d. During its intrathoracic course it is enclosed by the pericardium

27. **Lung**
    a. The right lung has three lobes and the left lung two lobes
    b. Blood is supplied to the lungs from the right ventricle via the pulmonary veins
    c. The horizontal fissure separates the two lobes of the left lung
    d. The pulmonary artery is the most superior component of the hilum of the left lung

28. **Abdominal wall**
    a. The neurovascular bundle runs between the layers of external oblique muscle (EOM) and internal oblique muscle (IOM)
    b. Transversalis fascia lies deep to the muscular layer
    c. The anterior abdominal wall muscles are innervated by the superior and inferior epigastric nerves
    d. The rectus sheath contains the superior and inferior epigastric arteries

29. **Testis, epididymis and spermatic cord**
    a. The venous system of the right testicle drains into the right renal vein
    b. The testicles' arterial supply arises from the internal iliac artery
    c. The testicles drain into the para-aortic lymph nodes
    d. The scrotum drains into the inguinal lymph nodes

30. **Small intestine**
    a. The duodenum is a retroperitoneal structure and is divided into three sections
    b. The duodenum receives its blood supply from the inferior mesenteric artery
    c. Meckel's diverticulum is a congenital anomaly which, when inflamed, can mimic appendicitis
    d. Sympathetic stimulation increases gut motility

31. Spleen
a. This is an extraperitoneal structure
b. It is associated posteriorly with the ninth to eleventh left ribs, and normally does not descend inferior to the costal region
c. Splenic rupture may be managed conservatively
d. The spleen enlarges into the left iliac fossa

32. Liver and portal circulation
a. The portal vein arises from the inferior mesenteric and splenic veins
b. There are four sites of portosystemic anastomosis
c. The liver drains via the hepatic veins to the inferior vena cava
d. The liver has a dual blood supply from the portal artery and hepatic artery

33. Rectum and anus
a. The rectum starts at the level of the third sacral vertebra (S3) as a continuation of the sigmoid colon
b. The pectinate line indicates the junction of the superior and inferior parts of the anal canal
c. The region superior to the pectinate line is extremely sensitive to pain
d. Damage to the spongy urethra results in a high riding prostate

34. Thyroid gland
a. This is supplied by branches of the internal carotid artery
b. The external laryngeal branch of the superior laryngeal nerve is closely related to the superior thyroid vascular pedicle
c. It is attached to the cartilaginous tracheal rings between C5 and T1
d. Venous drainage is into the external jugular vein

35. Recurrent laryngeal nerve
a. This arises from the glossopharyngeal nerve
b. The left recurrent laryngeal nerve winds around the left subclavian artery
c. The right recurrent laryngeal nerve winds around the right subclavian artery
d. A hoarse voice may occur after thyroid surgery

36. Arterial supply of the face
a. The facial artery arises from the internal carotid artery
b. The facial artery ends at the lateral angle of the eye
c. The superficial temporal artery arises from the external carotid artery
d. The superficial temporal artery can easily be palpated anterior to the tragus of the ear

37. **Venous drainage of the face**
    a. The facial vein drains into the external jugular vein
    b. Venous blood can drain into the cavernous sinus, from the facial vein, via the superior ophthalmic vein
    c. Venous blood can drain into the pterygoid venous plexus, via the inferior ophthalmic and deep facial veins
    d. The facial veins arise from the angular vein

38. **Cervical sympathetic chain**
    a. Damage can result in Horner's syndrome
    b. This consists of three ganglia on each side
    c. It provides sympathetic innervation for the head, neck, thorax and abdomen
    d. It has acetylcholine as its postsynaptic neurotransmitter

39. **Larynx**
    a. This arises superior to the hyoid bone and blends with the trachea at the sixth cervical vertebra
    b. It consists of two single cartilages and two pairs of cartilage
    c. The intrinsic laryngeal muscles alter the size and shape of the laryngeal inlet and also move the vocal folds
    d. The intrinsic laryngeal muscles are all supplied by the recurrent laryngeal nerve

40. **Oculomotor nerve**
    a. The nucleus lies in the pons
    b. It passes through the medial wall of the cavernous sinus
    c. It supplies superior, medial and inferior rectus and superior oblique muscles
    d. A complete lesion results in a constricted pupil

41. **Trigeminal nerve**
    a. It has motor and sensory functions
    b. The sensory component has three branches: ocular, maxillary and mandibular
    c. The bodies of the sensory fibres form the geniculate ganglion
    d. It forms part of the corneal reflex

42. **Facial nerve**
    a. Damage to the facial nerve can result in hyperacusis
    b. It transmits taste sensation from the posterior third of the tongue and the soft palate
    c. It is the motor supply to the muscles of facial expression
    d. A lower motor neuron lesion of the facial nerve results in paralysis of the muscles in the lower face with sparing of the upper face

43. **Cranial nerves IX (glossopharyngeal), X (vagus), XI (accessory) and XII (hypoglossal)**
    a. Cranial nerve IX supplies parasympathetic innervation to the thorax and abdomen
    b. Cranial nerve X innervates movement of the soft palate
    c. The vagus nerve transmits information from the receptors in the carotid body and carotid sinus
    d. Cranial nerves IX, X, XI and XII exit the cranium via the foramen magnum

44. **Cerebral blood supply**
    a. The anterior cerebral arteries supply the lateral aspects of the cerebral hemispheres
    b. The internal carotid artery gives off the anterior, middle and posterior cerebral arteries
    c. The anterior and posterior circulations are connected via the posterior cerebral artery
    d. The circle of Willis creates an anastomosis between the two hemisphere circulations

45. **Midbrain and posterior circulation**
    a. The midbrain lies predominantly in the middle cranial fossa
    b. The midbrain lies anterior to the tentorium cerebelli
    c. It is supplied by the middle cerebral artery
    d. It contains the dopaminergic cells of the substantia nigra

46. **Cerebrospinal fluid (CSF)**
    a. CSF is produced by the choroid plexus
    b. This drains via the cerebral aqueduct from the lateral ventricles to the third ventricle
    c. The total volume of the CSF is 1000–1500 mL
    d. The CSF drains from the fourth ventricle into the subarachnoid space

47. **Optic nerve**
    a. A lesion in the optic radiation results in a bitemporal hemianopia
    b. A lesion in the optic chiasma results in a homonymous hemianopia
    c. Lesions in the occipital lobe can result in macular sparing
    d. Lesions in the optic nerve result in monocular visual loss

48. **Vertebral column**
    a. There are seven cervical, twelve thoracic, five lumbar and five sacral vertebrae
    b. The pedicles connect the vertebral body to the transverse processes
    c. The laminae connect the spinous processes to the transverse processes
    d. The ligamentum flavum connects the posterior aspects of the vertebral bodies

49. Spinal cord

a. In adults the spinal cord extends to about the first or second lumbar vertebra
b. The bundle of nerve roots in the lumbar cistern caudal to the termination of the spinal cord is called the cauda equina
c. The epidural space lies between the dura and subarachnoid meningeal layers
d. The spinal subarachnoid space is a continuation of the subarachnoid space in the posterior fossa

50. Spinal tracts

a. The dorsal column transmits pain and temperature
b. The spinothalamic tract transmits vibration and position sense
c. The corticospinal tract transmits motor fibres
d. Hemisection of the spinal cord results in an ipsilateral loss of motor, proprioception and vibration sensation, with contralateral loss of pain and temperature sensation

I. Anatomy: Answers

Ia. F
Ib. T
Ic. T
Id. F
The lateral and medial pectoral nerves supply pectoralis major. The accessory nerve (cranial nerve XI) also supplies sternocleidomastoid. The long thoracic nerve supplies serratus anterior, paralysis of which results in winging of the scapula. Latissimus dorsi inserts into the intertubular groove of the humerus. It extends, adducts and medially rotates the humerus.

2a. F
2b. T
2c. F
2d. T
The muscles that make up the rotator cuff are supraspinatus, infraspinatus, subscapularis and teres minor. They all work together to keep the humeral head in the glenoid fossa. Supraspinatus and the deltoid muscle abduct the arm at the glenohumeral joint, infraspinatus and teres minor externally rotate the arm, and subscapularis internally rotates the arm. The rotator cuff is deficient inferiorly. Supraspinatus and infraspinatus are supplied by the suprascapular nerve.

3a. T
3b. T
3c. F
3d. T
The terminal branches of the brachial artery are the radial and ulnar arteries. This division occurs at the inferior border of the cubital fossa.

4a. T
4b. T
4c. T
4d. F
The lateral epicondyle is the common origin of the tendons for the extensor muscles of the forearm. The medial epicondyle is the common origin of the flexor muscles of the forearm.

5a. F
5b. F
5c. T
5d. F
The trochlea of the humerus articulates with the trochlear notch of the ulna. The capitulum articulates with the head of the radius. The lateral collateral ligament extends from the lateral epicondyle of the humerus and blends distally with the annular ligament of the radius. Ulnar nerve, rather than

median nerve, damage is a more frequent complication with avulsion fractures of the medial epicondyle as the nerve runs in close proximity to its posterior aspect. The ulnar nerve may also be injured in posterior dislocations of the elbow.

6a. T
6b. T
6c. F
6d. T
The common interosseous artery arises from the ulnar artery. It divides almost immediately into the anterior and posterior interosseous arteries. The ulnar artery enters the hand superficially above flexor retinaculum between pisiform and the hook of hamate.

7a. F
7b. T
7c. F
7d. F
Injuries to the superior aspect of the brachial plexus are often called Erb's palsy. Damage to the lower brachial plexus (C8 and T1) may be referred to as Klumpke's palsy. The muscles affected by Erb's palsy are biceps, brachialis, brachioradialis and deltoid. Supinator is supplied by the radial nerve, which arises from C7. The arm is medially rotated and the elbow extended but the shoulder adducted.

8a. T
8b. T
8c. T
8d. T
The blood supply to the scaphoid is from the distal end so a fracture through the waist of the scaphoid results in avascular necrosis of the proximal fragment.

9a. T
9b. T
9c. T
9d. T
Quadriceps femoris consists of vastus lateralis, vastus intermedius, vastus medialis and rectus femoris; they work together as one and are involved in extending the knee joint. Psoas major is supplied by the ventral rami of L1–3.

10a. F
10b. T
10c. T
10d. T
The inguinal ligament forms the superior aspect of the femoral triangle, the medial side of sartorius forms the lateral side, and the lateral side of adductor longus forms the medial side.

11a. T
11b. T
11c. F
11d. F
The sciatic nerve arises from L4 and L5 and S1−3. The sciatic nerve lies in the inferior inner quadrant of the buttocks so intramuscular injections must be given in the upper outer quadrant of the buttocks to avoid damage to the nerve. The sciatic nerve is more commonly damaged in posterior dislocation of the hip than in anterior dislocations. The sciatic nerve divides, in the popliteal fossa, into the common peroneal nerve and the tibial nerves.

12a. F
12b. T
12c. F
12d. T
The lateral superior border of the popliteal fossa is formed by the long head of biceps femoris, and the inferior borders consist of the two gastrocnemius heads. The superior medial border of the popliteal fossa is formed by semimembranosus, not semitendinosus. The sciatic nerve divides at the superior aspect of the popliteal fossa into the common peroneal (fibular) and tibial nerves. The common peroneal nerve then passes along the superior lateral aspect of the popliteal fossa to the head of the fibula, which it winds around before passing into the leg.

13a. T
13b. T
13c. F
13d. T
The posterior compartment of the lower leg is divided into a deep compartment and a superficial compartment, both of which are supplied by the tibial nerve and the posterior tibial artery. The superficial compartment contains gastrocnemius, soleus and plantaris, not popliteus. The deep compartment contains flexor hallucis longus, flexor digitorum longus, tibialis posterior and popliteus. The superficial and deep muscle groups are both enclosed in strong fascia; this region is therefore at high risk of compartment syndrome.

14a. F
14b. T
14c. T
14d. T
The deep branch of the common peroneal nerve, not the anterior tibial nerve, supplies the anterior compartment of the lower leg.

15a. T
15b. F
15c. T
15d. F
The tendons of peroneus longus and brevis pass posteriorly to the lateral malleolus. In inversion injuries of the ankle, the tuberosity of the base of the

fifth metatarsal may be avulsed by the peroneus brevis tendon. The lateral compartment of the lower leg is supplied by the superficial branch of the common peroneal nerve. The lateral compartment does not have an artery: the muscles are supplied superiorly by perforating branches of the anterior tibial artery and inferiorly by perforating branches of the fibular artery, which arises from the posterior tibial artery.

16a. T
16b. T
16c. F
16d. F
The medial aspect of the ankle joint is supported by the very strong deltoid ligament. The lateral ligament consists of three parts (anterior talofibular ligament, posterior talofibular ligament and calcaneofibular ligament), which are easily damaged in inversion injuries of the ankle joint. Dorsiflexion and plantarflexion occur at the ankle, and inversion and eversion at the subtalar joint. The ankle joint is more stable in dorsiflexion than plantar flexion because the body of the talus is wider anteriorly.

17a. F
17b. T
17c. T
17d. T
The common peroneal nerve (CPN) supplies the anterior and lateral muscular compartments of the lower leg. It arises from the sciatic nerve in the superior aspect of the popliteal fossa; it then winds around the lateral aspect of the fibular head. As the CPN winds around the head of the fibula, it is exposed and easily damaged. The resulting CPN palsy leads to foot drop. The loss of sensation is variable because a large part of this region is supplied by the sural nerve, which receives fibres from the tibial nerve as well as the CPN.

18a. T
18b. F
18c. F
18d. T
The superficial and deep peroneal nerves arise from the common peroneal nerve. The superficial branch transmits sensation from the dorsum of the foot and all digits, except the adjoining sides of the first and second digits, which are supplied by the deep peroneal nerve, and the lateral side of the fifth digit, which is supplied by the sural nerve. The saphenous nerve arises from the femoral nerve. It supplies the skin on the medial side of the leg and foot, as far anteriorly as the head of the first metatarsal. The sural nerve is formed by fibres from the common peroneal and tibial nerves. It transmits sensation from the skin on the posterior and lateral aspects of the leg and lateral side of the foot. The tibial nerve gives rise to the medial and lateral plantar nerves. The medial branch transmits sensation from the medial side of the sole of the foot and sides of the first three digits. The lateral branch supplies the sole lateral to the middle of the fourth digit. The skin of the heel is supplied by branches of the tibial and sural nerves. Knowledge of this anatomy is very helpful when it comes to performing nerve blocks at the ankle.

19a. T
19b. F
19c. T
19d. T
The spring ligament, also known as the plantar calcaneonavicular ligament, is a broad thick band of fibres that connects the sustentaculum tali of the calcaneus to the inferior/plantar surface of the navicular bone.

20a. F
20b. F
20c. T
20d. F
The first rib is the shortest and widest of all the ribs. It articulates with the first thoracic vertebra (T1), not C7. The first rib is well protected and so is fractured only in high-force incidents. The scalene anterior muscle arises from the transverse processes of the C3–6 vertebrae and attaches to the scalene tubercle on the superior surface of the first rib. The first rib lies in closed proximity to some very important structures:

- The subclavian vein, which passes over the first rib anteriorly to scalenus anterior muscle
- The brachial plexus
- The subclavian artery, which passes superiorly over the rib behind the scalenus anterior muscle.

21a. F
21b. F
21c. F
21d. T
The diaphragm is innervated by the phrenic nerves, which arise from C3–5. It has three main openings. The aortic opening is at the level of the inferior border of the T12 vertebra. This opening is a defect in the posterior aspect of the diaphragm so blood flow through the aorta is not affected by movements of the diaphragm during respiration. The aortic opening also allows the passage of the thoracic duct and sometimes the azygos vein. The oesophageal opening is at T10 and, unlike the aortic opening, it is in the diaphragmatic musculature. It therefore acts as a sphincter on the oesophagus when the diaphragm contracts. The inferior vena caval opening lies at the level of the T8–9 intervertebral disc.

22a. F
22b. T
22c. F
22d. F
The trachea arises at the level of C6. It divides into the right and left main bronchus at the carina (T4–5). The right main bronchus runs more vertically than the left main bronchus. This anatomical difference is important because it means that inhaled foreign bodies are more likely to lodge in the right main bronchus. The trachea is supported by horseshoe-shaped, incomplete rings of cartilage. The only complete ring of cartilage in the trachea is the cricoid

cartilage; this is why the cricoid ring is used to compress the oesophagus, during induction of anaesthesia, when there is a risk of aspiration.

23a. T
23b. F
23c. F
23d. T
The parietal and visceral layers of the serous pericardium comprise a sac surrounding the heart, in the same way that the pleurae surround the lungs. The pericardial cavity created by these layers contains serous fluid that allows the heart to beat without any friction. The fibrous pericardium is a tough structure that prevents overexpansion of the heart. The problem with this lack of flexibility is that, if the pericardial sac fills with fluid, the heart is unable to beat effectively (tamponade).

24a. T
24b. T
24c. T
24d. T
The surface anatomy of the heart is as follows:

- Right border: third right costal cartilage to the sixth right costal cartilage
- Inferior border: inferior end of the right border to the fifth intercostal space in the midclavicular line on the left
- Superior border: line between the inferior border of the second left costal cartilage to the superior border of the third right costal cartilage
- Left border: left end of the superior and inferior borders.

25a. T
25b. T
25c. F
25d. F
Murmurs associated with the pulmonary valve are best heard in the region along the left-hand edge of the upper sternal border, whereas murmurs associated with the aortic valve are best heard in the region on the right side of the upper sternum.

26a. F
26b. F
26c. T
26d. F
The oesophagus arises at C6 and ends at T10. It lies posteriorly to the left main bronchus and passes through the diaphragm at the level of T10 to join the stomach. It runs through the thorax on the anterior aspect of the vertebral bodies.

27a. T
27b. F
27c. F
27d. T

The right lung has three lobes. The horizontal fissure separates the upper and middle lobes and the lower lobe is separated from the rest of the right lung by the oblique fissure. The oblique fissure separates the two lobes of the left lung. The pulmonary arteries deliver blood from the right ventricle to the hila of the lungs. The hilum of the left lung consists of the pulmonary artery superiorly and the left main bronchus posteriorly, with the two pulmonary veins lying anteriorly and inferiorly to the left main bronchus. The right hilum has the right main bronchus in the posterior superior aspect, the two pulmonary arteries in the anterior region, and the pulmonary veins in the inferior portion.

28a. F
28b. T
28c. F
28d. T

The neurovascular bundle runs between the IOM layer and the transverse abdominis muscle (TAM). The abdominal wall consists of six layers: skin, subcutaneous tissue (superficial layer: Camper's fascia; deep layer: Scarpa's fascia), muscle, transversalis fascia, extra abdominal fat and parietal peritoneum. The anterior abdominal wall muscles are supplied by the thoracoabdominal nerve, and subcostal, iliohypogastric and ilioinguinal nerves.

29a. F
29b. F
29c. T
29d. T

The venous system of the left testicle drains to the inferior vena cava (IVC), via the left renal vein, whereas the right drains directly into the IVC. The testicles receive their blood supply from the aorta via the testicular arteries. This pattern is the result of the embryonic derivation of the testicles.

30a. F
30b. F
30c. T
30d. F

The duodenum is a retroperitoneal structure divided into four regions. It receives its blood supply from the superior mesenteric artery, which supplies the gastrointestinal tract from the insertion of the bile duct into the duodenum to the distal third of the transverse colon. Meckel's diverticulum is an anomaly that occurs in 1–2% of people. It is always on the antimesenteric border of the ileum and is usually located approximately 37 cm from the ileocaecal junction in infants and 50 cm in adults. It has the potential for inflammation, ulceration and perforation. In general, sympathetic stimulation reduces motility of the intestine and acts as a vasoconstrictor, thereby reducing or stopping digestion.

31a. F
31b. T
31c. T
31d. F
The spleen is entirely surrounded by peritoneum except at the hilum where the splenic branches of the splenic artery and vein enter and leave. The relations of the spleen are:

- Anteriorly the stomach
- Posteriorly the left part of the diaphragm
- Inferiorly the left colic flexure
- Medially the left kidney.

Repair of a ruptured spleen is difficult because the capsule is so thin; consequently, splenectomy is performed to prevent exsanguination. In some cases contained rupture may be managed conservatively. When the spleen enlarges, it extends into the right iliac fossa.

32a. F
32b. T
32c. T
32d. F
The portal vein arises from the superior mesenteric and splenic veins. Portosystemic anastomoses are the sites where the portal venous system communicates with the systemic venous system:

- One site is between the oesophageal veins and the azygos vein (systemic system), or the left gastric vein (portal system); when dilated these are oesophageal varices.
- There is an anastomosis between the rectal veins: the inferior and middle rectal veins drain into the IVC (systemic system), and the superior rectal veins continue as the inferior mesenteric vein (portal system).
- The paraumbilical veins of the anterior abdominal wall (portal system) form an anastomosis with the superficial epigastric veins (systemic system); when dilated these veins produce caput medusae.
- Twigs of colic veins (portal system) anastomose with retroperitoneal veins (systemic system).

The liver receives blood from the hepatic artery and portal vein; it then drains from the liver via the hepatic vein into the IVC.

33a. T
33b. T
33c. F
33d. F
The anal canal superior to the pectinate line differs from the inferior part in its arterial supply, innervation, and venous and lymphatic drainage as a result of its embryonic origins. The region superior to the dentate line is insensitive to pain, because it is supplied by autonomic nerves, whereas inferior to the dentate line the region is very sensitive to pain because it is supplied by the

inferior anal nerve, which contains sensory fibres. Damage to the intermediate part of the urethra results in a high riding prostate.

34a. F
34b. T
34c. T
34d. F
The thyroid gland is supplied by the superior and inferior thyroid arteries. The superior thyroid artery is a branch of the external carotid artery, and the inferior thyroid artery is a branch of the thyrocervical trunk, which arises from the subclavian artery. The thyroid gland consists of two lobes connected by the isthmus. The superior and middle thyroid veins drain into the internal jugular vein, and the inferior thyroid vein drains directly into the brachiocephalic vein.

35a. F
35b. F
35c. T
35d. T
The recurrent laryngeal nerve arises from the vagus nerve in the inferior part of the neck. On the right side the nerve loops around the right subclavian artery at T1−2 before ascending in the tracheo-oesophageal groove to the larynx. On the left side it loops around the arch of the aorta at T4−5. The nerve lies deep to the thyroid gland, often in close relationship to the inferior thyroid artery. Damage to one recurrent laryngeal nerve results in paralysis of the ipsilateral vocal fold. This presents with a weak, hoarse voice.

36a. F
36b. F
36c. T
36d. T
Most facial arteries arise from the external carotid artery at the angle of the mandible. The artery runs inside the mandible until half-way along the body, when it passes under the inferior edge. It then continues superiorly past the angle of the mouth to the medial angle of the eye. The facial artery gives off branches to the upper and lower lips and the lateral side of the nose. The superficial temporal artery ascends anterior to the ear to the temporal region and ends in the scalp by dividing into the frontal and parietal branches. It emerges on the face between the temporomandibular junction (TMJ) and the ear.

37a. F
37b. T
37c. T
37d. T
The facial vein arises at the medial angle of the eye, as a continuation of the angular vein. The facial vein ends by draining into the internal jugular vein. At the medial angle of the eye, the facial vein communicates with the superior ophthalmic veins. These veins also drain into the cavernous sinus. Inferior to the margin of the mandible, the facial vein is joined by the anterior branch of

the retromandibular vein. The retromandibular vein also drains into the pterygoid venous plexus. These two connections are very important, because any infection in the triangular area from the upper lip to the bridge of the nose can spread, via these valveless veins, intracranially.

38a. T
38b. T
38c. F
38d. F
Presynaptic autonomic nerve fibres arise in the brain. They pass down the spinal cord and exit via the anterior root. They then pass via the white ramus communicans to the sympathetic ganglia, which lie alongside the spine. In the ganglion the presynaptic nerve transmits information to the postsynaptic nerve using acetylcholine as the neurotransmitter. The postsynaptic nerve then exits the ganglion via the grey rami communicantes and passes to the target organ, where noradrenaline (norepinephrine) is released. Only the ganglia of T1–L2 receive white rami directly.

The cervical sympathetic chain has three ganglia. The superior cervical ganglion lies at the level of C1–2. It supplies sympathetic innervation to the cranial cavity, via the internal and external carotid artery plexus, the superior four cervical spinal nerves and the cardiac plexus. The middle cervical ganglion lies at C6; it supplies innervation for the C5 and C6 spinal nerves and the cardiopulmonary splanchnic nerve and fibres to the thyroid gland via the periarterial plexus. The inferior cervical ganglion (C7–T1) provides fibres for the seventh and eighth cervical spinal nerves, the inferior cervical cardiac nerve and the periarterial nerve plexus. This plexus surrounds the vertebral artery and supplies more fibres to the cranial cavity.

Horner's syndrome results from damage to the sympathetic chain and results in miosis (pupillary constriction), ptosis and anhidrosis (lack of facial sweating on the ipsilateral side).

39a. F
39b. F
39c. T
39d. F
The larynx arises inferior to the hyoid bone but does blend with the trachea at the level of C6. It consists of single and paired cartilages, joints, ligaments and membranes. Of the cartilages, three are single – thyroid, cricoid and epiglottic – and three are paired – arytenoids, corniculate and cuneiform. The laryngeal muscles are functionally divided into the intrinsic and extrinsic groups. The extrinsic laryngeal muscles move the larynx as a whole. The infrahyoid muscles are depressors of the hyoid bone and larynx whereas the suprahyoid and stylopharyngeus muscles are elevators of the hyoid bone and larynx. The intrinsic laryngeal muscles move the laryngeal parts. All but one of the intrinsic muscles are supplied by the recurrent laryngeal nerve. The cricothyroid muscle is supplied by the external laryngeal nerve, which is a branch of the superior laryngeal nerve.

40a. F
40b. F
40c. F
40d. F
The oculomotor nucleus lies in the midbrain. After emerging from the midbrain the nerve pierces the dura and runs in the lateral wall of the cavernous sinus. It enters the orbit though the superior orbital fissure. The oculomotor nerve supplies four of the six extraocular muscles – superior rectus, medial rectus, inferior rectus and inferior oblique – as well as levator palpebrae superioris. The superior oblique muscle is the only muscle supplied by the trochlear nerve (IV). The oculomotor nerve also carries parasympathetic fibres to the ciliary muscle, for pupil accommodation, and sphincter pupillae, for constriction of the pupil. A complete lesion of the oculomotor nerve results in pupil dilatation as a result of interruption of the parasympathetic supply.

41a. T
41b. F
41c. F
41d. T
The trigeminal nerve arises from a small motor nucleus in the pons and a large sensory nucleus, which spans a large portion of the brain stem. The motor part supplies the muscles of mastication. The bodies of the sensory fibres form the trigeminal ganglion, not the geniculate ganglion, which is part of cranial nerve VII. The sensory component has three divisions: ophthalmic (V1) maxillary (V2) and mandibular (V3). The mandibular branch also carries the motor fibres. The corneal reflex (blinking in response to the cornea being touched) is created by the trigeminal nerve, which carries the afferent fibres, and is completed by the facial nerve, which carries the efferent fibres.

42a. T
42b. F
42c. T
42d. F
The facial nerve emerges from the junction of the pons and medulla. It has two divisions; the larger motor root innervates the muscles of facial expression whereas the smaller root carries taste via the chorda tympani from the anterior two-thirds of the tongue and soft palate, parasympathetic fibres to the sublingual and submandibular salivary gland, and sensory fibres that transmit sensation from a small area of skin around the external acoustic meatus. Sensation from the posterior third of the tongue is transmitted by the glossopharyngeal nerve. In its route it passes though the posterior cranial fossa, internal acoustic meatus, facial canal, stylomastoid foramen and parotid gland, where it divides into its terminal branches. An upper motor neuron lesion rather than a lower motor neuron lesion results in sparing of the forehead. This occurs because there is dual innervation of the forehead. The facial nerve supplies stapedius, and therefore damage to the nerve results in paralysis of stapedius, which causes hyperacusis (an oversensitivity to sound).

43a. F
43b. T
43c. F
43d. F

The glossopharyngeal nerve transmits parasympathetic fibres to the parotid glands and the glands in the posterior third of the tongue. The glossopharyngeal nerve transmits taste sensation from the posterior third of the tongue as well as general sensation from the tongue and pharynx. It also has a motor branch, which supplies stylopharyngeus. It is the glossopharyngeal nerve that transmits information from the carotid sinus and carotid body. The vagus nerve, along with other functions, provides parasympathetic fibres to the chest and thorax, and motor innervation to the muscles of the soft palate and intrinsic laryngeal muscles. The accessory nerve has cranial and spinal roots. The cranial root provides motor innervation to the soft palate and pharynx, and the spinal root innervates trapezius and sternocleidomastoid. The hypoglossal nerve innervates the muscles of the tongue. Cranial nerves IX–XII exit the cranium via the jugular foramen.

44a. F
44b. F
44c. F
44d. T

The cerebral blood supply is divided into two components: the anterior circulation, which arises from the internal carotid artery, and the posterior circulation, which arises from the vertebral and basilar arteries. The internal carotid artery arises from the common carotid artery in the neck. It enters the cranial cavity via the carotid canal and cavernous sinus. The terminal branches of the internal carotid artery are the anterior and middle cerebral arteries. The anterior cerebral artery supplies the medial aspect of the hemispheres, whereas the middle cerebral artery supplies the lateral aspect except for the occipital lobe. The two anterior cerebral arteries are connected via the anterior communicating artery. The anterior circulation is connected to the posterior circulation via the posterior communicating arteries.

45a. F
45b. T
45c. F
45d. T

The midbrain lies predominately in the posterior cranial fossa. The edge of the tentorium cerebelli lies on its dorsal surface. The posterior circulation, which arises from the vertebral and basilar arteries, supplies the occipital lobes, cerebellum and brain stem. The vertebral arteries join at the level of the caudal border of the pons to form the basilar artery. The basilar artery ends by dividing into the two posterior cerebral arteries. The posterior cerebral arteries supply the inferior surface of the brain, occipital pole and midbrain. The midbrain is also supplied by the superior cerebellar arteries, which arise from the basilar artery. The pons is supplied by the pontine branches and the cerebellum by the anteroinferior and superior cerebellar arteries, all of which arise from the basilar arteries. The cerebellum also receives blood supply from the posteroinferior cerebellar artery, which arises bilaterally from the vertebral arteries. The medulla is supplied by the posteroinferior cerebellar arteries and branches of the vertebral and basilar arteries.

46a. T
46b. F
46c. F
46d. T
CSF is produced by the choroid plexus. The bulk of the CSF is produced in the lateral ventricles although there is also choroid plexus in the third and fourth ventricles. The CSF drains from the lateral ventricles via the interventricular foramina into the third ventricle. It then drains through the cerebral aqueduct into the fourth ventricle, from where it drains via a single median aperture and paired lateral apertures into the subarachnoid space. The foramina in the fourth ventricle are the only routes of exit for the CSF; if these become obstructed CSF accumulates and the ventricles distend, producing compression of the cerebral hemispheres. The CSF is reabsorbed via the arachnoid villi into the dural venous system. The total volume of CSF is 100–150 mL. About 500–750 mL CSF is produced per day.

47a. F
47b. F
47c. T
47d. T
The optic nerve arises from the eyeball. It exits the orbit via the optic canal and enters the middle cranial fossa, where it forms the optic chiasma. It is in the chiasma that fibres from the nasal half of each retina cross over and join the temporal fibres from the other side to form the optic tracts. It is as a result of this crossing of fibres in the chiasma that lesions in this region cause a bitemporal hemianopia (loss of vision of half of the visual field in both eyes). Most fibres in the optic tract then terminate in the lateral geniculate bodies. Lesions in the optic tract result in loss of the temporal fibres on the same side as the lesion and nasal fibres on the contralateral side (homonymous hemianopia). From the lateral geniculate bodies the fibres pass to the visual cortices of the occipital lobes in the optic radiation. Macular sparing occurs in occipital lobe lesions as a result of the dual blood supply to the region (posterior cerebral and middle cerebral arteries).

48a. T
48b. T
48c. T
48d. F
The ligamentum flavum connects the adjacent vertebral arches together by attaching to the laminae.

49a. T
49b. T
49c. F
49d. T
The epidural (extradural) space is the space between the periosteum-lined bony wall of the vertebral canal and the dura mater.

50a. F
50b. F
50c. T
50d. T
The dorsal (posterior) column transmits vibration and proprioception. These fibres travel in the ipsilateral half of the spinal cord. They synapse in the medulla, then cross the midline and continue to the thalamus. The spinothalamic tract transmits pain and temperature sensation. These fibres cross to the contralateral side almost as soon as they enter the spinal cord.

2. Physiology: Questions

1. **Regarding negative feedback systems that act to maintain homeostasis**
   a. The negative feedback system consists of detectors, comparators and effectors
   b. The 'set point' is a wide range of variables around which the effectors act
   c. The 'set point' is fixed once adulthood is reached
   d. Effectors act to move the variable in the opposite direction to the change that was originally detected

2. **Fluid distribution in the body**
   a. Water accounts for approximately 30% of body mass
   b. Sixty-five per cent of body water exists within the extracellular space, which includes the plasma and fluid between cells
   c. Potassium concentration is higher in the intracellular fluid than in plasma
   d. Most of the body's sodium is located within the cells

3. **Regarding the cell**
   a. It is the smallest functional unit of a living organism
   b. The genetic material is contained within the nucleus
   c. It is contained within a membrane that consists entirely of proteins
   d. Mitochondria convert adenosine triphosphate to adenosine diphosphate for use as energy within the cell

4. **The Na^+/K^+ ATPase pump**
   a. This binds three sodium (Na^+) ions internally and two potassium (K^+) ions externally
   b. The carrier protein is phosphorylated by 10 ATP molecules, changing its conformation
   c. Sodium is pumped into the cell and potassium out of the cell down a diffusion gradient
   d. Drugs that act on the Na^+/K^+ pump include digoxin and omeprazole

5. **Flow through a tube is directly affected by the following**
   a. The viscosity of the fluid
   b. The diameter of the tube
   c. The length of the tube
   d. The pressure differences across the end of the tube

6. Respiration is controlled by the following
   a. CO_2 receptors in the carotid body
   b. The Hering–Breuer reflex
   c. The pH of CSF
   d. Respiratory centres in the cerebellum

7. Regarding lung function tests
   a. The residual volume is the volume of air remaining in the lungs after normal expiration
   b. The FEV_1/FVC ratio typically reduces in obstructive airway disease
   c. The normal tidal volumes in a healthy adult are 10 mL/kg
   d. The total lung capacity can be measured using a spirometer

8. The Hb/O_2 dissociation curve
   a. This shifts to the right in the presence of fever
   b. It shifts to the left as pH decreases: the Bohr effect
   c. Fetal Hb has an increased affinity for O_2
   d. It shifts to the left in carbon monoxide poisoning

9. Pulmonary vascular resistance is increased by the following
   a. Hypocapnia
   b. Hypoxia
   c. Acidosis
   d. Adrenaline (epinephrine)

10. 2,3-DPG concentration in red blood cells is increased
    a. In the presence of anaemia
    b. In cyanotic congenital heart disease
    c. In blood stored for transfusion
    d. In trained athletes

11. Cyanosis
    a. This appears more readily in anaemic patients
    b. It is marked in patients with cyanide poisoning
    c. It may be seen without significant hypoxia in the presence of polycythaemia
    d. It remains despite supplemental oxygen in congenital heart disease with a right-to-left shunt

12. Airway resistance is increased by the following
    a. With increased respiratory rate
    b. By vagal stimulation
    c. If inhaled carbon dioxide levels rise
    d. With increased circulating adrenaline (epinephrine) levels

13. **Total oxygen delivery to tissues**
    a. It normally equates to the rate of oxygen consumption
    b. Normally >98% of oxygen transported is combined with haemoglobin
    c. It falls by half if the haemoglobin concentration is halved
    d. It doubles if oxygen consumption doubles

14. **In the investigation of respiratory disease**
    a. Perfusion scans use ^{133}Xe
    b. Gas transfer factor usually increases in severe emphysema
    c. Gas transfer factor usually decreases in pulmonary embolism
    d. Gas transfer factor measures the thickness of the alveolar membrane

15. **The following shift the oxygen dissociation curve to the left**
    a. Sickle cell disease
    b. Hyperpyrexia
    c. Acidosis
    d. Hypercapnia

16. **Phaeochromocytomas**
    a. These are typically benign tumours of the adrenal cortex
    b. They are commonly bilateral
    c. They most commonly cause sustained hypertension
    d. They release noradrenaline (norepinephrine), adrenaline (epinephrine) and dopamine

17. **Carbon dioxide in blood**
    a. In a compensated metabolic acidosis, $PaCO_2$ is raised
    b. Most is in the form of bicarbonate
    c. Haemoglobin buffers the H^+ generated by carriage of CO_2
    d. For any given pH, the $PaCO_2$ is inversely proportional to the bicarbonate concentration

18. **Lung volumes**
    a. After normal expiration the lungs contain about 3 litres of air
    b. The normal dead space in an adult is about 500 mL
    c. The functional residual capacity is more than the residual volume
    d. The residual volume is about 1.5 litres in a healthy adult

19. **Partial pressure CO_2 in arterial blood**
    a. This increases during sleep
    b. It is raised at high altitudes
    c. It decreases in response to metabolic acidosis
    d. It is raised in type 1 respiratory failure

20. **At high altitude**
    a. Pulmonary vascular resistance falls
    b. Hyperventilation occurs
    c. 2,3-DPG levels decrease
    d. Renal bicarbonate excretion decreases

21. **In the cardiovascular system**
    a. The total blood volume is approximately 7% of the fat-free body mass
    b. Approximately 80% of the blood circulates on the arterial side of the system
    c. The kidneys receive approximately 5% of the cardiac output
    d. The blood pressure in the pulmonary circulation is less than that of the systemic circulation

22. **In cardiac physiology**
    a. Cardiac output is equal to the heart rate multiplied by the systolic blood pressure ($CO = HR \times SBP$)
    b. The cardiac output is increased during exercise by an isolated increase in heart rate
    c. The pulse pressure is the difference between the systolic and diastolic blood pressures ($PP = SBP - DBP$)
    d. The mean arterial pressure is equal to the diastolic pressure plus half of the systolic pressure ($MAP = DBP + \frac{1}{2}SBP$)

23. **The coronary circulation**
    a. This receives approximately 4% of the total cardiac output
    b. It is not affected by cardiac contractions
    c. It is maximal during diastole
    d. The left and right coronary arteries are branches from the arch of the aorta

24. **During the cardiac cycle**
    a. The closure of the mitral valve occurs when the pressure in the left atrium is greater than the pressure in the left ventricle
    b. At rest atrial contraction is responsible for over 80% of ventricular filling
    c. The first heart sound coincides with the closure of the aortic valve
    d. The mean end-diastolic volume in the left ventricle is approximately 50 mL

25. **The following ECG changes and parts of the cardiac cycle are correctly paired**
    a. P wave – atrial depolarisation
    b. QRS complex – ventricular repolarisation
    c. Q–T interval – overall time for depolarisation and repolarisation of the ventricles
    d. T wave – atrial repolarisation

26. **The following leads of the ECG and voltage changes are correctly paired**
    a. Lead I – voltage between the left and right arms
    b. Lead II – voltage between the right arm and right leg
    c. Lead III – voltage between the left arm and left leg
    d. Lead IV – voltage between the left and right legs

27. **Cardiac oxygen consumption**
    a. This is decreased in patients with hypertension
    b. It is greater when the ventricular pressure is high and the stroke volume low, than when the ventricular pressure is low and the stroke volume high
    c. It is increased with physical exercise
    d. It can be estimated using the Fick principle

28. **The following are potent vasoconstrictors of the peripheral circulation**
    a. Endothelin-1
    b. Histamine
    c. Acetylcholine
    d. Angiotensin II

29. **Regarding substance exchange across capillaries**
    a. Oxygen and carbon dioxide are hydrophilic and diffuse easily across the cell membrane
    b. Diffusion of hydrophilic substances is quicker than that of lipophilic substances
    c. Glucose crosses the capillary wall mainly via gaps between endothelial cells
    d. A reduction in plasma proteins will cause an increase in filtration and a loss of fluid into the tissues

30. **The circulation of skeletal muscle**
    a. This receives, at rest, approximately 20% of cardiac output
    b. It has increased blood flow during exercise due to the release of potassium and calcium
    c. It has a minimal effect on total peripheral resistance
    d. It is largely responsible for thermoregulation

31. **Regarding special circulations**
    a. The pulmonary circulation is controlled by autonomic nerves
    b. Arteriovenous anastomoses, mainly in the skin of the hands, feet and face, allow blood flow directly into the venous plexus and facilitate heat loss as part of thermoregulation
    c. An increase in $PaCO_2$ reduces cerebral blood flow
    d. The coronary circulation extracts about 70% of the oxygen of the blood flowing through it

32. In the stomach
a. Hydrochloric acid secretion from parietal cells occurs predominantly in the cardia
b. Acid secretion is increased by histamine
c. Intrinsic factor from chief cells is vital for vitamin B_{12} absorption
d. NSAIDs predispose to peptic ulceration by increasing acid secretion

33. Liver
a. This receives approximately 10% of cardiac output via the portal vein and hepatic artery
b. It is the major source of erythrocyte production in the fetus
c. It synthesises glycogen from fat, carbohydrate and amino acids
d. It synthesises coagulation factors V, VII, IX and X

34. In the digestion of protein
a. Pepsin is inactivated by the acidic environment within the stomach
b. The action of pepsin on protein produces dipeptides
c. Trypsin activates chymotrypsin and elastase
d. Amino acids are absorbed using a Na^+ co-transport mechanism

35. Iron
a. Most dietary iron is in the ferrous form
b. Absorption occurs mainly in the terminal ileum
c. Co-ingestion of ascorbic acid aids iron absorption
d. It binds to transferrin in intestinal epithelial cells

36. Bile acids
a. These act as detergents
b. They are synthesised from bilirubin and biliverdin
c. They undergo extensive reabsorption in the gut
d. When they reach the colon they cause diarrhoea

37. In the pancreas
a. The pancreatic secretions are slightly acidic
b. Secretin stimulates pancreatic enzyme release
c. Trypsinogen is converted to active trypsin as it mixes with bile in the pancreatic duct
d. Trypsin activates trypsinogen

38. Gut motility
a. Gallbladder contraction is induced by cholecystokinin
b. Sympathetic stimulation increases the activity of intestinal smooth muscle
c. The parasympathetic supply to the anal sphincter is inhibitory
d. The internal anal sphincter is controlled via the pudendal nerve

39. Diarrhoea
    a. Cholera causes inflammatory diarrhoea
    b. Secretory diarrhoea occurs following an ileal resection
    c. *Shigella* causes an inflammatory diarrhoea
    d. *E. coli* enterotoxins cause a secretory diarrhoea

40. Secretin
    a. This is excreted from the stomach
    b. Secretion is increased by acid in the duodenum
    c. It causes relaxation of the pyloric sphincter
    d. Secretion is inhibited by somatostatin

41. Regarding the kidney
    a. The kidney receives approximately 20% of the cardiac output
    b. Each kidney contains approximately 10 000 nephrons
    c. There are three types of nephron
    d. The kidneys have no endocrine function

42. In patients with the following arterial blood gas results
    a. pH < 7.35: high $PaCO_2$ and normal base excess = respiratory acidosis
    b. pH < 7.35: normal $PaCO_2$ and negative base excess = metabolic acidosis
    c. pH > 7.45: low $PaCO_2$ and normal base excess = respiratory alkalosis
    d. pH > 7.45: normal $PaCO_2$ and positive base excess = metabolic alkalosis

43. Regarding the loop of Henle
    a. Fluid entering the descending limb is hyperosmolar when compared with plasma
    b. The thin descending limb is impermeable to urea, but permeable to water
    c. The ascending limb is impermeable to urea, but permeable to water
    d. There is passive diffusion of Na^+ and Cl^- into the thick ascending limb

44. Pituitary gland
    a. It lies above the ethmoid sinus
    b. The posterior lobe is formed together with the hypothalamus
    c. The anterior lobe secretes ADH
    d. It lies between the cavernous sinuses

45. The adrenal cortex secretes the following
    a. Testosterone
    b. Angiotensin
    c. Noradrenaline (norepinephrine)
    d. Aldosterone

46. **Aldosterone**
    a. It is a polypeptide hormone
    b. It is secreted in response to a fall in blood volume
    c. It acts to increase renal artery pressure
    d. It increases sodium reabsorption

47. **Adrenaline (epinephrine)**
    a. It is secreted from the adrenal cortex in response to stress
    b. It decreases the peripheral vascular resistance
    c. It causes pupillary constriction
    d. It promotes glycogenolysis in skeletal muscle

48. **Hypoadrenalism**
    a. This may present with cardiovascular collapse
    b. It results in hypernatraemia
    c. It is associated with a metabolic acidosis
    d. It is usually due to primary adrenal failure

49. **Secondary hypoadrenalism**
    a. This is associated with severe electrolyte abnormalities
    b. It results from adrenal suppression by exogenous steroids
    c. It is associated with pigmentation of the buccal mucosa
    d. It may follow head injury

50. **Hyperkalaemia**
    a. This leads to elevated aldosterone levels
    b. It stimulates renin release
    c. It inhibits glucagon release
    d. It stimulates insulin release

2. Physiology: Answers

1a. T
1b. F
1c. F
1d. T
Homoeostasis is a process of physiological self-regulation that maintains steady states within the body through coordinated physiological activity. The negative feedback system operates around a narrow range of variables called the set point, which can vary throughout life. The term 'negative feedback' applies when the effectors move in the opposite direction to the change detected and thus have a negative effect on the variable.

2a. F
2b. F
2c. T
2d. F
Water makes up 50–70% of body mass. Most of this (about 65%) is within the cells in the intracellular fluid (ICF). The balance between the ICF and extracellular fluid (ECF) is tightly controlled, because many physiological processes depend upon its composition. The composition of the different fluid spaces with regard to ionic concentration is listed below (TBW is total body water).

	ECF (35% TBW) (mmol/L)		
	Interstitial fluid (22%)	Plasma (13%)	ICF (65% TBW) (mmol/L)
Sodium (Na^+)	143	143	10
Potassium (K^+)	4	4	140
Calcium (Ca^{2+})	3	3	<0.01
Chloride (Cl^-)	129	108	3–30
Bicarbonate (HCO_3^-)	29	29	9

3a. T
3b. T
3c. F
3d. F
The cell is the smallest functional unit of a living organism: a cell is able to perform essential vital functions such as metabolism, growth, movement, reproduction and hereditary transmission. The cell membrane consists of lipids with membrane proteins (allowing the movement in and out of cells) or ions and proteins. Mitochondria enable the synthesis of adenosine triphosphate via the citric acid cycle and the respiratory chain.

4a. T
4b. F
4c. F
4d. T
The Na^+/K^+ ATPase pump acts to maintain the cellular environment and move solutes and ions against their concentration gradient. The process requires the carrier protein to be phosphorylated by one ATP molecule. Diffusion is a passive process, not requiring the consumption of ATP, whereas the Na^+/K^+ pump is an example of active transport.

5a. T
5b. T
5c. T
5d. T
The flow of any liquid through a tube is dependent on the pressure across the ends of the tube and the resistance within. The resistance is calculated using Poiseuille's law and includes the viscosity of the fluid, and radius and length of the tube. The radius of the tube is the most important component with the resistance being proportional to the radius to the power of 4 (flow $\propto r^4$).

6a. F
6b. T
6c. T
6d. F
Respiration is controlled by respiratory centres, which are in the pons and medulla. Inputs are received from chemoreceptors in the carotid body sensing O_2 and central chemoreceptors in the medulla responding to a rise in CO_2 and consequent pH drop. Pulmonary stretch receptors send input to the respiratory centre via the vagus nerve (the Hering–Breuer reflex).

7a. F
7b. T
7c. F
7d. F
Normal tidal volume is about 500 mL (7 mL/kg). Vital capacity is the air expired after maximal inspiration. Residual volume is the air remaining after maximum expiration. Spirometry does not measure residual volume; gas dilution techniques are therefore needed to measure total lung capacity.

Dynamic lung function tests measure forced expiratory volume in 1 second (FEV_1) and forced vital capacity (FVC). In obstructive diseases FEV_1/FVC reduces; in restrictive conditions it increases.

8a. T
8b. F
8c. T
8d. T
The Hb/O_2 dissociation curve, when shifted to the right (a decreased affinity for oxygen), releases oxygen more readily to metabolically active tissue. Shifts to the right occur with raised CO_2, raised 2,3-DPG (2,3-diphosphogycerate),

raised temperature and lowered pH (Bohr effect). Dissociation curve shifts to the left (an increasing affinity for oxygen) occur with fetal Hb (enhancing placental oxygen uptake), decreased CO_2, decreased temperature, decreased 2,3-DPG and increased pH. The presence of carbon monoxide increases the affinity of Hb for oxygen but does not release it to the tissues.

9a. F
9b. T
9c. T
9d. T
Raised CO_2 leads to decreased pH and vasoconstriction. Constricting vessels in areas of low oxygen shunts blood away from under-ventilated alveoli.

10a. T
10b. T
10c. F
10d. F
2,3-DPG, generated by glycolysis, binds to Hb, reducing the affinity of Hb for oxygen, and shifting the dissociation curve to the right (oxygen is more readily released to the tissues). Levels fall rapidly in stored blood, reducing the oxygen delivery capacity. 2,3-DPG levels rise in response to hypoxia, high altitude, hypocapnia, alkalosis and anaemia. Levels transiently increase after exercise.

11a. F
11b. F
11c. T
11d. T
Cyanosis is visible when >5 g/dL reduced Hb is present; with anaemia the total Hb is low. Conversely, in polycythaemia modest reductions in oxygen may produce cyanosis. Cyanide, by inhibiting cytochrome oxidase, leads to a failure of oxygen utilisation by the tissues; the oxygen content in the blood remains high and arterialisation of venous blood occurs. In conditions where a significant shunt occurs within the lungs, either anatomical or functional, supplemental oxygen fails to enter the circulation.

12a. T
12b. T
12c. F
12d. F
Raised respiratory rate leads to increasing turbulent flow, increasing airway resistance. Parasympathetic vagal stimulation, via increasing bronchial muscle tone and increasing secretions, increases resistance. Sympathetic stimulation via β_2-adrenergic receptors causes bronchial smooth muscle relaxation. Raised inhaled CO_2 leads to bronchodilatation.

13a. F
13b. T
13c. F
13d. F
Oxygen delivery is a function of cardiac output, Hb level and saturation. At rest, oxygen consumption is approximately 250 mL/min, with about 25% of the total oxygen delivered. Approximately 1.5% of oxygen is dissolved, most being delivered bound to Hb. When Hb levels fall oxygen delivery to tissues is maintained by a compensatory increase in cardiac output. The extraction ratio increases when consumption increases, e.g. during exercise.

14a. F
14b. F
14c. T
14d. F
Ventilation scans use inhaled xenon and perfusion scans use radioactive technetium. Gas transfer factor is a measure of how efficiently oxygen is transferred from the alveolus to the red blood cell. It is elevated in asthma, pulmonary haemorrhage, polycythaemia and left-to-right shunts.

15a. F
15b. F
15c. F
15d. F
All shift the dissociation curve to the right. For a given partial pressure of oxygen there is a decreased affinity of Hb for oxygen; i.e. the Hb 'gives up' oxygen more easily to the tissues.

16a. F
16b. F
16c. T
16d. T
Phaeochromocytomas are tumours of the adrenal medulla (90%); 10% are bilateral and 10% occur outside the adrenal glands, usually being paraganglionic in the organ of Zuckerkandl next to the aortic bifurcation. Most cause sustained hypertension, although only 0.1% of hypertensive patients will be found to have a phaeochromocytoma. Approximately 15% of tumours will release catecholamines episodically, producing palpitations, headache, glycosuria and hypertension. Pure adrenaline-secreting tumours, via stimulation of β_2-receptors causing peripheral vasodilatation, may mimic septic shock.

17a. F
17b. T
17c. T
17d. F
$PaCO_2$ (partial arterial pressure of CO_2) is lowered in the respiratory compensation of metabolic acidosis.

CO_2 is predominantly carried in the blood as bicarbonate:

$$CO_2 + H_2O \rightarrow HCO_3^- + H^+$$

$PaCO_2$ is proportional to the bicarbonate concentration:

$PaCO_2 = pH \times \kappa \times HCO_3^-$ (where κ = dissociation coefficient of carbonic acid).

18a. T
18b. F
18c. T
18d. T
The functional residual volume is the volume remaining in the lungs after quiet expiration, equal to approximately 3 litres in an adult. The dead space is normally about 150 mL. The residual volume is the gas remaining after maximal expiration, and the functional residual capacity is the residual volume plus the expiratory reserve volume.

19a. T
19b. F
19c. T
19d. F
The partial pressure of CO_2 in arterial blood rises during periods of hypo-ventilation, as occurs during sleep. Conversely, in hypoxic environments (as at high altitude), hyperventilation lowers arterial CO_2.

Respiratory compensation of metabolic acidosis lowers CO_2. Type 1 respiratory failure, hypoxic respiratory failure, results in hyperventilation; CO_2 is lowered. It is raised in type 2 respiratory failure.

20a. F
20b. T
20c. F
20d. F
At high altitude, the acute response to the hypoxic environment is pulmonary vasoconstriction. Peripheral chemoreceptors trigger hyperventilation, which reduces arterial CO_2. Central chemoreceptors, because of the increase in pH, act to reduce the drive to hyperventilation. This is overcome by metabolic compensation over 2–3 days with an increase in renal excretion of bicarbonate. Over a longer time course, to improve oxygen carriage, 2,3-DPG levels increase and polycythaemia occurs.

21a. T
21b. F
21c. F
21d. T
The total blood volume is approximately 7% of the fat-free body mass, which is roughly 4–5 litres in the adult. Most of the circulation at any one time is in the low-pressure venous side of the circulation. The kidneys receive 20% of the total cardiac output. The pulmonary circulation is at a much lower pressure than that of the arterial circulation.

22a. F
22b. F
22c. T
22d. F
In clinical practice it is essential to know some simple physiological equations:

Cardiac output = heart rate × stroke volume:

$$CO = HR \times SV$$

Pulse pressure = systolic blood pressure − diastolic blood pressure:

$$PP = SBP - DBP$$

Mean arterial pressure = diastolic blood pressure + ⅓systolic pressure:

$$MAP = DBP + \tfrac{1}{3}SBP$$

The MAP uses one-third of the value of the SDP, as the heart spends approximately 60% of the time in diastole.

During exercise the CO is increased by an increase in both HR and SV.

23a. T
23b. F
23c. T
23d. F
The coronary circulation arises from the root of the aorta, with the left coronary artery supplying the left ventricle and the right coronary artery supplying the right ventricle in most individuals. The amount of blood flow to cardiac muscle varies throughout the cardiac cycle and is maximal in diastole, although these pressure effects are less pronounced in the right ventricle where the overall pressure is less.

24a. F
24b. F
24c. F
24d. F
Valvular closure during the cardiac cycle occurs when the pressure in the distal area is greater than that in the proximal area: the mitral valve closes when the pressure in the left ventricle exceeds that in the left atrium, and the aortic valve closes when the pressure in the aorta is greater than that in the left ventricle. At rest, atrial contraction contributes only approximately 20% of final ventricular volume − most filling occurs as a result of venous pressure. The mean end-diastolic volume in the left ventricle is approximately 120 mL − 70 mL of this will form the stroke volume and 50 mL will be left in the ventricle (the end-systolic volume).

25a. T
25b. F
25c. T
25d. F
Knowledge of the different parts of an ECG (electrocardiogram) and how they relate to cardiac function is vital in everyday emergency medicine:

- P wave: atrial depolarisation
- QRS complex: ventricular depolarisation
- Q–T interval: time for depolarisation and repolarisation of the ventricles
- T wave: ventricular repolarisation
- U wave: repolarisation of the Purkinje fibres.

26a. T
26b. F
26c. T
26d. F
Einthoven's triangle is formed by leads I, II and III (there is no lead IV). The limb leads are placed on the left and right arms, and the left leg. Lead I is the voltage between the left and right arms, lead II is the voltage between the right arm and left leg, and lead III is the voltage between the left arm and left leg.

27a. F
27b. T
27c. T
27d. T
Cardiac oxygen consumption and myocardial oxygen demand increase with cardiac output. Therefore anything that increases the cardiac output will increase cardiac oxygen consumption. Oxygen demand is greater when the ventricular pressure is high and the stroke volume small than when the ventricular pressure is low and the stroke volume high, even though the same amount of work is performed. Therefore patients with hypertension (where the ventricular pressure is high) have an increased cardiac oxygen demand. The Fick principle can be used to estimate cardiac output and cardiac oxygen consumption.

28a. T
28b. F
28c. F
28d. T
Vasoconstrictors act by binding to receptors and causing a rise in intracellular calcium (Ca^{2+}). Potent vasoconstrictors include noradrenaline (norepinephrine), endothelin-1, angiotensin, antidiuretic hormone (vasopressin) and thromboxane. Endogenous substances that cause vasodilatation include histamine, nitric oxide, substance P, bradykinin, acetylcholine and prostaglandins D_2 and E_2.

29a. F
29b. F
29c. T
29d. T
The capillary endothelial lipid bilayer can be crossed easily by substances that are lipophilic, such as oxygen and carbon dioxide. Hydrophilic substances cross the membrane much more slowly, often via gaps in the endothelial wall. Decrease of oncotic pressure exerted by plasma proteins causes increased filtration and movement of fluid into tissues. This is seen clinically in patients with a loss of proteins (e.g. proteinuria in nephritic syndrome) or a decrease in protein production (e.g. liver cirrhosis), with development of peripheral oedema as a result of fluid accumulation.

30a. T
30b. F
30c. F
30d. F
Skeletal muscle receives at rest approximately 20% of cardiac output, with many of its capillaries not being perfused. Blood flow increases greatly during exercise to as much as 80% of the cardiac output, with capillaries being recruited by the release of potassium and carbon dioxide from muscle (metabolic hyperaemia). Skeletal muscle is a large contributor to total peripheral resistance, but the skin performs most of the body's thermoregulatory functions.

31a. F
31b. T
31c. F
31d. T
The pulmonary circulation is controlled mainly by hypoxic pulmonary vasoconstriction, with little or no input from autonomic nerves or metabolic products. An increase in $PaCO_2$ causes cerebral vasodilatation and therefore increases cerebral blood flow. Due to its high oxygen demand, the coronary circulation has developed to extract a high proportion of the oxygen in the blood flowing through it.

32a. F
32b. T
32c. F
32d. F
Acid production in the stomach occurs from parietal cells, predominantly in the body with few in the cardia. Secretion is increased by gastrin, acetylcholine and histamine. Intrinsic factor is from parietal calls; chief cells produce pepsinogen.

NSAIDs (non-steroidal anti-inflammatory drugs) inhibit cyclooxygenase, and so reduce prostaglandin secretion, decreasing mucus and bicarbonate secretion.

33a. F
33b. T
33c. F
33d. T
The liver receives approximately 25% of the cardiac output. During fetal development (in months 2–7 of gestation, ceasing before birth) the liver is an erythropoietic organ.

The liver synthesises glycogen from carbohydrate and amino acids only. Hepatic production of clotting factors V, VII, IX, X and prothrombin occurs.

34a. F
34b. F
34c. T
34d. T
Pepsin initiates protein digestion, activated by the acidic pH within the stomach. It produces polypeptides. Trypsin also activates phospholipase A_2, co-lipase and carboxypeptidase. Amino acids are absorbed via a secondary active transport system within the duodenum and jejunum. Sodium and amino acids bound to a carrier enter cells down a sodium gradient. Na^+/K^+ ATPase pumps the sodium out again (primary active transport).

35a. F
35b. F
35c. T
35d. F
Most dietary iron is in the ferric (Fe^{3+}) form, which is reduced to the ferrous (Fe^{2+}) form by ascorbic acid/ferriductase before absorption in the duodenum. Iron binds to transferrin in plasma and binds to ferritin in enterocytes, particularly if intake exceeds requirements. The excess is shed by epithelial desquamation.

36a. T
36b. F
36c. T
36d. T
Bile acids act as detergents, emulsifying lipids. They are predominantly synthesised from cholesterol. The primary bile acids are conjugated with glycine or taurine to increase solubility. Intestinal bacteria convert these into secondary bile acids, of which 95% are reabsorbed, mainly from the terminal ileum, via the enterohepatic circulation to return to the liver. Excess bile salts reaching the colon produce secretory diarrhoea.

37a. F
37b. F
37c. F
37d. T
Pancreatic exocrine secretions are very alkaline, rich in bicarbonate. Secretin acts on the pancreas to secrete pancreatic juice and stimulate bile secretion.

Cholecystokinin (CCK) acts on the acinar cells to release zymogen granules, secreting a low-volume, high-enzyme content juice.

Trypsinogen is converted to active trypsin in the duodenum by the brush border enzyme enteropeptidase. Trypsin autocatalyses trypsinogen, and the release of trypsin within the pancreas would lead to autodigestion of the organ.

38a. T
38b. F
38c. T
38d. F
Parasympathetic, cholinergic activity increases gut motility; sympathetic, nor-adrenergic activity decreases motility and causes sphincter contraction. The internal anal sphincter is under involuntary control, and the sympathetic supply is excitatory, parasympathetic and inhibitory. The external sphincter is under voluntary control via the pudendal nerve.

39a. F
39b. T
39c. T
39d. T
Diarrhoea results from four mechanisms. Osmotic diarrhoea occurs when non-absorbed hypertonic substances are present in the lumen. Secretory forms are seen with enterotoxins (e.g. cholera and *Escherichia coli*) and the presence of colonic bile salts or fatty acids, as occurs after ileal resection. Mucosal destruction causes inflammatory diarrhoea as seen in dysentery (*Shigella*) and inflammatory bowel disease. Abnormal motility caused by dia-betes or hyperthyroidism, or post-vagotomy may produce diarrhoea.

40a. F
40b. T
40c. F
40d. T
Secretin is secreted by S-cells in the mucosa of the upper small intestine. It is excreted in response to acid and protein in the duodenum. It acts to increase excretion of the highly alkaline pancreatic secretions, which in turn neutralise duodenal contents, reducing secretin production. Secretin acts to decrease stomach acid secretion and close the pyloric sphincter.

41a. T
41b. F
41c. F
41d. F
The kidney receives approximately 20% of the cardiac output. Each kidney has approximately 10^6 nephrons, of which there are two types: the cortical nephrons, which have glomeruli in the outer aspect of the cortex and short loops of Henle, and the juxtamedullary nephrons, the glomeruli of which lie close to the cortex medullary boundary and have long loops of Henle. The

kidney has an endocrine function, producing hormones including renin, erythropoietin and prostaglandins.

42a. T
42b. T
42c. T
42d. T
The ability to evaluate correctly the acid–base status of a patient is a vital everyday skill in emergency medicine. A normal pH lies between 7.35 and 7.45.

43a. F
43b. T
43c. F
43d. F
The fluid that enters the loop of Henle via the descending limb is isotonic with plasma, and the high osmolality that is generated in the medulla depends upon active transport of ions in the thick ascending limb, the countercurrent multiplier, and differential permeabilities to water and solutes in different regions. The thin descending limb is permeable to water but impermeable to urea. The ascending limb is impermeable to water and permeable to urea. The mechanism for reabsorption of Na^+ and Cl^- is active and requires the $Na^+/K^+/2Cl^-$ co-transporter.

44a. F
44b. T
44c. F
44d. T
The pituitary gland is composed of two lobes, a posterior lobe formed from the diencephalic forebrain, together with the hypothalamus, and an anterior lobe derived from ectoderm. The gland lies in the pituitary fossa of the sphenoid bone, above the sphenoid sinus, and between the cavernous sinuses, containing the internal carotid arteries.

45a. F
45b. F
45c. F
45d. T
The adrenal glands comprise two parts: the cortex and the medulla. Cortical hormones include glucocorticoids (cortisol, corticosterone) from the zona fasiculata, mineralocorticoids (aldosterone) from the zona glomerulosa, and androgens (dehydroepiandrosterone and androstenedione) from the zona reticularis. Adrenal androgens are converted peripherally to testosterone. The adrenal medulla secretes adrenaline (epinephrine), noradrenaline (norepinephrine) and dopamine.

46a. F
46b. T
46c. T
46d. T
Aldosterone, like all adrenal cortex hormones, is derived from cholesterol precursors. It is secreted from the adrenal cortex in response to angiotensin II and raised potassium. It acts on the renal tubule to reabsorb sodium and chloride and consequently water, increasing ECF volume and blood pressure. It is part of the renin–angiotensin system: renal juxtaglomerular cells secrete renin in response to a decreased perfusion pressure, decreased sodium or sympathetic stimulation. Renin activates angiotensinogen (produced in the liver) to angiotensin I. Angiotensin-converting enzyme (ACE) in the lung and kidney converts angiotensin I to angiotensin II, which acts to increase aldosterone secretion.

47a. F
47b. T
47c. F
47d. T
Adrenaline (epinephrine), secreted from the adrenal medulla in response to stress, acts on the liver and skeletal muscle to promote glycogenolysis, increasing glucose levels and mobilising free fatty acids. It raises the metabolic rate and elevates plasma lactate. Via α-receptors it causes mydriasis.

48a. T
48b. F
48c. T
48d. F
Hypoadrenalism is most commonly caused by withdrawal of steroid medication. Addison's disease, primary adrenal failure, occurs as a result of destruction of the glands by autoimmune processes, infection, infiltration or infarction. Primary hypoadrenalism also tends to destroy the adrenal cortex, causing loss of mineralocorticoids. This causes hyponatraemia, hyperkalaemia and raised hydrogen ion concentrations. The associated dehydration of adrenal failure causes an elevated urea. Hypoadrenalism may be insidious and chronic, and result in a significant postural drop in blood pressure or complete cardiovascular collapse.

49a. F
49b. T
49c. F
49d. T
Secondary hypoadrenalism occurs by either suppression of the gland from exogenous steroids (as little as 7.5 mg prednisolone per day) or failure of ACTH production. ACTH (adrenocorticotrophin) levels are low, so there is no abnormal pigmentation, as seen in Addison's disease. The zona glomerulosa is intact, mineralocorticoids remain functional, and therefore the biochemical abnormalities seen with primary hypoadrenalism are absent. Secondary hypoadrenalism follows pituitary failure of any cause, including head trauma, tumours and Sheehan's syndrome.

50a. T
50b. F
50c. F
50d. T
Elevated potassium levels directly stimulate the release of aldosterone and inhibit renin release by acting on the macula densa. Potassium promotes the release of both insulin and glucagon from the pancreas.

3. Pharmacology: Questions

1. **In NSAID-associated ulceration**
   a. Adverse effects from NSAIDs are rare
   b. Prostaglandins (PGE_2 and PGI_2) increase gastric acid secretion
   c. Eradication of *Helicobacter pylori* will reduce the risk of NSAID-induced bleeding
   d. Ibuprofen is less likely to cause serious gastrointestinal side effects than diclofenac

2. **Adenosine**
   a. This has a half-life of approximately 10 min
   b. It is a naturally occurring purine nucleoside
   c. It is useful in the management of supraventricular and ventricular arrhythmias
   d. It is the drug of choice to cardiovert patients with tachycardias related to Wolff–Parkinson–White syndrome

3. **Mannitol**
   a. This should be given to all patients with head injury and a reduced GCS
   b. It is a loop diuretic similar in action to furosemide
   c. It decreases cerebral blood flow by reducing blood viscosity and microcirculatory resistance
   d. It may produce renal failure or hypotension if given in large doses

4. **β Blockers**
   a. They are all water soluble
   b. They should never be used in patients with diabetes
   c. They are used in the treatment of heart failure, migraine and hypothyroidism
   d. They should never be used in combination with digoxin

5. **Regarding some of the β blockers**
   a. Propranolol is a non-selective β blocker with a half-life of 3–6 hours
   b. Esmolol has a rapid onset of action and short half-life, and is useful in the treatment of ventricular arrhythmias
   c. Sotalol is not recommended for the treatment of angina or hypertension
   d. Labetalol has an arterial vasodilating action

6. Regarding the renin–angiotensin system

a. Renin is released from the juxtaglomerular apparatus in the kidney

b. Renin acts on angiotensin I, converting it into angiotensin II

c. Angiotensin II is a powerful vasoconstrictor of arterioles

d. Angiotensin-converting enzyme is found primarily in the blood vessels of the lungs

7. ACE inhibitors such as captopril and enalapril

a. These are useful in the treatment of hypertension, heart failure and angina

b. They should not be used in patients with renal artery stenosis or hypokalaemia

c. They may cause cough due probably to a potentiation of the action of bradykinin

d. They may cause first-dose hypotension, especially in those on diuretics

8. In the treatment of angina

a. The main aim is to reduce the work of the heart and therefore its oxygen demand

b. Glyceryl trinitrate (GTN) acts by producing nitrous oxide (N_2O), which causes peripheral vasodilatation in the venous system

c. Patients on longer-acting nitrates may develop tolerance that can be reduced by introducing a nitrate-free period of 4–8 hours each day

d. GTN should be avoided in patients with aortic regurgitation

9. Calcium channel blockers

a. These act only on one site and therefore have a limited therapeutic use

b. They block L-type voltage-sensitive channels in arteriolar smooth muscle

c. They cause vasoconstriction and increase preload

d. They can all be safely used with β blockers

10. Regarding treatment of cardiac arrest

a. Sodium bicarbonate is indicated in all causes of cardiac arrest where the arterial pH is <7

b. Regardless of pH, sodium bicarbonate should be given in cardiac arrest associated with hyperkalaemia or tricyclic antidepressant overdose

c. Calcium should be given during resuscitation from pulseless electrical activity (PEA) if it is thought to be caused by hypo-calcaemia, overdose of calcium channel-blocking drugs or hypokalaemia

d. The initial dose of calcium chloride when indicated is 10 mL 10%, which is 6.8 mmol Ca^{2+}

11. **Regarding antiplatelet agents**
    a. Aspirin has been shown to reduce mortality in patients who have had a myocardial infarction
    b. Aspirin reduces platelet aggregation by an inhibition of thromboxane A_2 formation
    c. Clopidogrel has a synergistic action when given with aspirin
    d. Clopidogrel should be given to all patients presenting with chest pain

12. **Thrombolytics in acute myocardial infarction**
    a. These should not be given to patients over the age of 75
    b. They inhibit the formation of plasmin
    c. They are not useful unless given within 30 min of the patient arriving in the emergency department
    d. The risk of haemorrhagic stroke is approximately 10%

13. **β_2 Agonists (such as salbutamol)**
    a. These may be given orally, subcutaneously, intravenously or by inhalation
    b. They may cause hyperkalaemia and should therefore be used with caution in patients on spironolactone
    c. They act by causing smooth muscle relaxation via an increase in intracellular cAMP
    d. They may commonly cause adverse effects such as fine tremor, tachycardia and hypotension

14. **Ipratropium bromide**
    a. This is an anticholinergic agent
    b. It is a derivative of atropine and has a maximum effect between 30 and 60 min
    c. Side effects include dry mouth, urinary retention and tachycardia
    d. It may interact with warfarin and cause lengthening of the INR

15. **Benzodiazepines**
    a. These act on NMDA receptors and cause an increase in intracellular calcium
    b. They may be the first-line treatment for seizures
    c. They are useful in the management of acute anxiety and should be considered for the long-term treatment of patients with sleep disturbance
    d. Their effects are reversed by naloxone

16. **Tricyclic antidepressants: actions at the following receptors cause the related side effects**
    a. Histamine receptors causing drowsiness and sedation
    b. Dopamine receptors causing dystonia and dyskinesia
    c. α-Adrenoreceptors causing hypertension
    d. Muscarinic receptors causing dry mouth, blurred vision and constipation

17. **Regarding vomiting**
    a. Emesis is coordinated by the vomiting centre, which is located in the pons
    b. The chemoreceptor trigger zone contains both dopamine receptors and $5HT_3$ receptors
    c. The use of metoclopramide is not recommended in males
    d. Cyclizine has its antiemetic effect by the blockade of dopamine receptors

18. **Morphine**
    a. This exerts many of its analgesic effects via actions at μ receptors
    b. In high doses it causes respiratory depression and mydriasis
    c. It should never be used as pain relief in patients who are addicted to heroin
    d. It can cause itching and flushing of the skin due to histamine release

19. **Regarding antiepileptic medication**
    a. Phenytoin probably achieves its action via blockade of K^+ channels
    b. Phenytoin is metabolised via a first-order process and is therefore safe in increased doses
    c. Sodium valproate should be avoided, if possible, in pregnant women
    d. Carbamazepine and phenytoin may exacerbate porphyria

20. **Penicillins**
    a. These are not useful agents in the treatment of Gram-positive infections
    b. They are bacteriostatic
    c. They act in the DNA of the bacterial cell
    d. They all may be given orally or intravenously

21. **Tetracyclines**
    a. These are usually the antibiotic of choice in urethritis, Q fever and Lyme disease
    b. They should not be used in children under the age of 12 years
    c. They are often given intravenously in severe infections
    d. They act by inhibiting bacterial protein synthesis

22. **The aminoglycoside antibiotics such as gentamicin**
    a. These are usually given orally
    b. They are most active against Gram-negative bacteria and are often used in life-threatening infections
    c. They should not be given to patients with renal dysfunction
    d. They require regular monitoring of serum levels to prevent toxicity

23. **The following are all used in the initial treatment of tuberculosis**
    a. Isoniazid
    b. Ribavirin
    c. Pyridoxine
    d. Ethambutol

24. **Which of the following infections are correctly paired with an appropriate antibiotic?**
    a. Meningitis: cefotaxime
    b. Lower urinary tract infection: ciprofloxacin
    c. Gonorrhoea: ciprofloxacin
    d. Typhoid fever: benzylpenicillin

25. **Insulin**
    a. This is secreted by the α cells of the islets of Langerhans in the pancreas
    b. It causes a rise in serum potassium
    c. It stimulates synthesis of glycogen by the liver
    d. It increases breakdown of lipids

3. Pharmacology: Answers

1a. F
1b. F
1c. F
1d. T

Adverse effects from NSAIDs (non-steroidal anti-inflammatory drugs) are common, especially as they are often given for long periods of time to elderly patients. NSAIDs inhibit cyclooxygenase and decrease the production of prostaglandins, which are protective, via a decrease in gastric acid secretion. Although eradicating *H. pylori* may help reduce the overall risk of ulceration in those starting long-term NSAID treatment that have dyspepsia or a history of ulceration, it is unlikely to reduce the risk of NSAID-induced bleeding or ulceration in those already on NSAIDs. Ibuprofen is the NSAID associated with the lowest risk of bleeding.

2a. F
2b. T
2c. F
2d. F

Adenosine is a naturally occurring purine nucleoside that has a half-life of approximately 10 seconds, so its side effects, such as dyspnoea and bronchospasm, are short-lived. It is useful in supraventricular tachycardia via its action at the AV (atrioventricular) node. In Wolff–Parkinson–White (WPW) syndrome, adenosine (and other AV node-blocking drugs such as calcium channel blockers, β blockers and digoxin) may cause a faster ventricular rate from unopposed and potentially enhanced conduction through an accessory pathway. This may degenerate in ventricular fibrillation.

3a. F
3b. F
3c. F
3d. T

Mannitol is an osmotic diuretic that may be useful in patients with deepening coma, pupil inequality or deterioration in neurological function. It is an osmotic diuretic that reduces cerebral oedema by preventing movement of water from the vascular space into the cells via the creation of an osmotic gradient. This reduces brain volume and may prevent herniation by allowing more space for swelling or an expanding haematoma. It also has other neuroprotective effects, promoting cerebral blood flow and scavenging free radicals.

4a. F
4b. F
4c. F
4d. F
Some β blockers are water soluble and some are lipid soluble. Those that are water soluble are less likely to enter the brain and therefore cause less sleep disturbance and nightmares. They can be used with caution in patients with diabetes, but may blunt their awareness of hypoglycaemia and cause deterioration in their glucose tolerance. They are useful in the treatment of many conditions including angina, heart failure, myocardial infarction, arrhythmias, thyrotoxicosis, anxiety, migraine and glaucoma. They should not be used with verapamil because this may cause severe hypotension, heart failure and asystole, but may be useful when combined with digoxin to control the ventricular rate in atrial fibrillation, especially when associated with thyrotoxicosis.

5a. T
5b. F
5c. T
5d. T
Propranolol is a non-selective β blocker that is now infrequently used in emergent settings as a result of the development of more cardioselective agents. Esmolol has a rapid onset, is short-acting and is used in the treatment of supraventricular arrhythmias. Labetalol has an arterial vasodilating action, but no advantages over other agents have been demonstrated in the treatment of hypertension.

6a. T
6b. F
6c. T
6d. T
Angiotensinogen is converted into angiotensin I (a 10 amino acid peptide cleaved from one end) by the action of renin. Angiotensin-converting enzyme (ACE) cleaves Angiotensin I into two amino acids including angiotensin II (an eight amino acid peptide). Angiotensin II acts in many ways to increase circulating volume, including increasing peripheral resistance and venous return to the heart, stimulating thirst, and increasing salt appetite, as well as the production of aldosterone and antidiuretic hormone (ADH).

7a. F
7b. F
7c. T
7d. T
ACE inhibitors are very useful drugs in a wide range of conditions, but have no role in the treatment of angina. Due to their action on the renin–angiotensin system, reducing the production of angiotensin II and aldosterone, patients are more likely to retain potassium and are at risk of developing hyperkalaemia. In patients with severe bilateral renal artery stenosis, ACE inhibitors may reduce or abolish glomerular filtration and are likely to cause severe and progressive renal failure.

8a. T
8b. F
8c. T
8d. F
Glyceryl trinitrate acts by the formation of nitric oxide (NO), which increases cGMP and causes vasodilatation. In patients with any form of outflow obstruction, such as severe aortic stenosis, there is a fixed afterload that is unaffected by drugs. Nitrates will cause a reduction in preload, which, in a patient with aortic stenosis, may compromise the cardiac output to such a degree that syncope may occur.

9a. F
9b. T
9c. F
9d. F
Calcium channel blockers differ in their attraction to different sites depending on the type of compound used; therefore they have a variation in therapeutic effect. They are useful in the treatment of angina, hypertension and cerebral vasospasm in aneurysmal subarachnoid haemorrhage. They cause relaxation of arteriolar smooth muscle and reduce afterload. Both verapamil and diltiazem affect conduction through the AV node and should be used with extreme caution in patients also taking β blockers.

10a. F
10b. T
10c. F
10d. T
The administration of sodium bicarbonate routinely during cardiac arrest and CPR (cardiopulmonary resuscitation), or even after the return of spontaneous circulation, is not recommended, but may be useful in the treatment of hyperkalaemia or tricyclic antidepressant overdose. Calcium is indicated in hyperkalaemia.

11a. T
11b. T
11c. T
11d. F
Aspirin prevents thomboxane A_2 formation by irreversibly inhibiting cyclooxygenase. This reduces the production of thromboxane A_2, which is a powerful inducer of platelet aggregation. Clopidogrel acts via a different mechanism from aspirin by blocking the effects of ADP on platelets. It has a relatively weak anti-platelet action on its own. Clopidogrel is indicated for the management of non-ST-elevation acute coronary syndrome in those with a moderate-to-high risk of myocardial infarction or death.

12a. F
12b. F
12c. F
12d. F
Until the advent of percutaneous angioplasty, treatment with thrombolytics was the mainstay of therapy for acute myocardial infarction. No trials have provided evidence to withhold treatment on the basis of patient's age alone, although there is an increased risk of haemorrhagic stroke in those aged over 75. Thrombolysis should be given as soon as the need for treatment is recognised, but may be beneficial up to 12 hours after symptom onset. The risk of haemorrhagic stroke is quoted in most papers at around 1%.

13a. T
13b. F
13c. T
13d. F
Salbutamol and other β_2 agonists are exceptionally effective treatments in patients with asthma. They may be given by multiple routes, but the most commonly used in the ED are inhaled, nebulised and intravenous injection. The β_2 agonists cause hypokalaemia via their sympathetic action on cells (salbutamol may be used as a treatment for hyperkalaemia). This sympathetic action is also responsible for its most common side effects: fine tremor, palpitations, tachycardia and nervous tension.

14a. T
14b. T
14c. T
14d. F
Ipratropium is often combined with β_2 agonists in the treatment of asthma. Its muscarinic anticholinergic action blocks parasympathetic bronchoconstriction and secretions, helping reverse acute airway obstruction. It is a quaternary derivative of atropine and shares the side effects common to all anticholinergic agents. Its effects are maximal within about 1 hour and last up to 6 hours.

15a. F
15b. T
15c. F
15d. F
The benzodiazepines act by directly enhancing GABA-mediated neuronal inhibition. GABA (γ-aminobutyric acid) binds to $GABA_A$-receptors and increases Cl^- conductance. Benzodiazepines bind to the GABA-receptor and, via a conformational change in the structure of the channel, increase Cl^- conductance and therefore neuronal inhibition. This inhibitory effect is useful in the management of seizures, and benzodiazepines are first-line drugs in their management in the ED. They may be useful for the short-term management of acute anxiety states but, due to the occurrence of dependence, even after short-term use, they should be used only in patients where insomnia is severe, disabling or causing extreme distress. The effects of benzodiazepines are reversed by flumazenil, but this should be used with caution in patients with

mixed overdose because it may potentiate the effects of other central nervous system stimulants taken concomitantly.

16a. T
16b. F
16c. F
16d. T
Tricyclic antidepressants block actions at histamine receptors causing drowsiness, α-adrenoreceptors causing postural hypotension and muscarinic receptors causing dry mouth, blurred vision, constipation and urinary retention. They have no actions at dopamine receptors. Although specific receptors and their pharmacology are not mentioned in the MCEM syllabus, some knowledge of the common receptor types will aid your ability to answer other questions.

17a. F
17b. T
17c. F
17d. F
Vomiting is coordinated by the vomiting centre, which is located in the medulla. This may be stimulated by the chemoreceptor trigger zone, which is located nearby. These areas have dopamine and serotonin or $5HT_3$-receptors; hence the use of dopamine receptor (D_2-receptor antagonists [such as metoclopramide and prochlorperazine], and $5HT_3$-receptor antagonists [such as ondansetron]) in the treatment of vomiting. Acute dystonic reactions are more commonly associated with the use of the D_2-receptor antagonists in young women and elderly people, and their routine use in these groups is not recommended. Cyclizine exerts its antiemetic effects via its action on histamine receptors.

18a. T
18b. F
18c. F
18d. T
Morphine is a highly effective analgesic that should be considered in patients with moderate-to-severe pain in the ED. It has actions at three different receptors, μ, χ and δ, but most of its analgesic action occurs via the μ receptors. In high dose it causes respiratory depression (via μ receptors) and miosis (via χ receptors). It is still useful in treatment of severe pain in patients with opiate addiction, but due to tolerance higher doses may be needed to have a satisfactory analgesia effect.

19a. F
19b. F
19c. T
19d. T
Phenytoin probably works by blocking the repetitive firing of neurons via deactivation of voltage-sensitive sodium channels. It is metabolised, similar to sodium valproate, by a zero-order process, meaning that blood levels may rise

disproportionately in relation to dose increments. This occurs when hepatic enzymes involved in its metabolism become saturated. Most of the antiepileptic medications, including carbamazepine, valproate and phenytoin, are teratogenic, and it is recommended that women wishing to become pregnant be informed of this risk and consult a specialist. Many drugs used regularly in emergency medicine practice may precipitate acute porphyria and the antiepileptics are among these.

20a. F
20b. F
20c. F
20d. F
The penicillins act by inhibiting the formation of peptidoglycan cross links during bacterial cell wall synthesis, allowing water into the cell and causing it to burst. As they kill the organism, they are bactericidal (bacteriostatic agents only inhibit bacterial growth). They are most useful in the treatment of Gram-positive infections such as those of staphylococci and streptococci (both Gram-positive cocci), diphtheria (a Gram-positive bacillus), and selected Gram-negative infections such as those of meningococci and gonococci (both Gram-negative cocci). Many penicillins are active orally and intravenously, but benzylpenicillin cannot be given orally because it is destroyed by gastric acid.

21a. T
21b. T
21c. F
21d. T
Tetracyclines remain useful antibiotics in a wide range of clinical conditions and are particularly indicated in infections caused by *Chlamydia* (urethritis), rickettsiae (Q fever), *Brucella* and the spirochaete *Borrelia burgdorferi* (the infecting agent in Lyme disease). As they bind to calcium in growing bones and teeth, they are not recommended in children under 12 years of age. They are usually given orally and none of the commonly used tetracyclines is available in intravenous form.

22a. F
22b. T
22c. F
22d. T
The aminoglycosides are highly effective antibiotics and are especially useful in the treatment of life-threatening Gram-negative infections. They are not active orally and must be given by injection. They can be given to patients with renal dysfunction, but the dose and interval between doses will have to be adjusted accordingly.

23a. T
23b. F
23c. F
23d. T
The four drugs used in the initial stages of treatment for tuberculosis are isoniazid, rifampicin, pyrazinamide and ethambutol. Ribavirin is an antiviral drug used in the treatment of respiratory syncytial virus. Pyridoxine is vitamin B$_6$ and, although sometimes used to prevent isoniazid neuropathy in those with pre-existing risk factors, it is not part of the treatment regimen for tuberculosis itself.

24a. T
24b. F
24c. T
24d. F
The recommended antibiotic treatment for lower urinary tract infection (UTI) is trimethoprim, nitrofurantoin, amoxicillin or an oral cephalosporin. Ciprofloxacin is indicated only in cases of acute pyelonephritis. The antibiotics of choice in typhoid fever are cefotaxime or ciprofloxacin.

25a. F
25b. F
25c. T
25d. F
Insulin is a 51 amino acid-containing polypeptide that is secreted from the β cells of the islets of Langerhans in the pancreas. It is released as a precursor called proinsulin, which is then hydrolysed to form insulin and C-peptide, in response to a rise in plasma glucose. Its actions include: uptake of glucose and its utilisation in fat and muscle cells; increased synthesis of glycogen and decreased formation of glucose in the liver; decreased lipid breakdown and increased protein synthesis; and increased uptake of potassium into cells (lowering serum potassium).

4. Microbiology: Questions

1. *Neisseria meningitidis* (**meningococcus**)
   a. It is always pathological to humans
   b. Immunisation is available against all the virulent strains
   c. It survives well outside the body
   d. It has a polysaccharide capsule

2. **Herpes simplex encephalitis**
   a. This shows a predilection for the occipital lobe
   b. It typically has a rapid symptom onset
   c. It is a mild self-limiting disease
   d. It is diagnosed by CSF PCR

3. **Concerning immunity**
   a. Immunity in newborns is the result of transplacental transfer of maternal T cells
   b. Elevated IgM signifies recent infection
   c. Defects in the complement pathway predispose to infections with *Neisseria* species
   d. Splenectomy predisposes to cryptococcal infections

4. **The following are notifiable diseases**
   a. HIV
   b. Malaria
   c. Food poisoning
   d. Chickenpox

5. **Regarding neutrophils**
   a. Most are found in the circulation
   b. Adhesion is mediated by opsonin
   c. A neutrophilia with left shift is due to the appearance of immature forms
   d. A neutrophilia occurs following exercise

6. **Miliary tuberculosis (TB)**
   a. This is diagnosed easily by examining sputum for acid-fast bacilli
   b. It is frequently diagnosed only at post-mortem examination
   c. It is highly contagious
   d. Lumbar puncture in meningeal TB usually shows elevated protein and glucose levels

7. Toxic shock syndrome
a. This results from a superantigen toxin
b. Over 80% of cases are associated with tampon use
c. It typically follows streptococcal infection
d. It is usually associated with a petechial rash

8. *Clostridium* spp.
a. These cause clinical effects by the release of endotoxins
b. They are spore-forming, anaerobic, Gram-negative bacilli
c. *Clostridium perfringens* causes gas gangrene and food poisoning
d. Symptomatic *Clostridium difficile* infection occurs only after antibiotic use

9. Malaria
a. Benign malaria is usually caused by *Plasmodium ovale*
b. It is excluded if no parasites are seen on a blood film
c. Malaria occurring in pregnancy is associated with a poorer prognosis
d. It may present more than 9 months after return from an endemic area

10. In the UK immunisation schedule
a. Diphtheria, tetanus and pertussis are given at 2, 3, 4 and 18 months of age
b. Pneumococcal vaccination is given at 2, 4 and 13 months
c. Chickenpox immunisation is given with the MMR immunisation
d. Tetanus and diphtheria vaccines are live attenuated vaccines

11. The following causative organisms and disease pairings are correct
a. *Borrelia burgdorferi* – Weil's disease
b. *Corynebacterium* sp. – diphtheria
c. Rhabdovirus – dengue fever
d. Rotavirus – bronchiolitis

12. Pelvic inflammatory disease (PID)
a. This usually results from the haematogenous spread of organisms
b. *Chlamydia* is the most frequent causative organism
c. When caused by gonorrhoea it may be accompanied by a perihepatitis
d. Treatment should be commenced only once the causative organism has been confirmed

13. Bacterial endocarditis
a. This is excluded by a negative blood culture
b. It is most commonly the result of staphylococcal infection
c. In intravenous drug users it is commonly due to *Strep. bovis*
d. It affects the tricuspid and pulmonary valve more often in injecting drug users

14. **Myocarditis is associated with infection with**
    a. HIV
    b. *Borrelia* spp.
    c. EBV
    d. *Strep. viridans*

15. **Viral meningitis**
    a. This is usually a mild, self-limiting disease
    b. It is most commonly caused by HSV-1 infection
    c. It occurs most commonly in winter
    d. Examination of the CSF shows a lymphocytosis

16. **The virulence of streptococci is increased by the following**
    a. Bacterial production of streptokinase
    b. The presence of cell surface G-proteins
    c. Being an encapsulated organism
    d. Bacterial production of Panton–Valentine leukocidin

17. **HIV/AIDS**
    a. AIDS is defined in the UK by a CD4 count <200
    b. Seroconversion occurs within 4 weeks of infection
    c. Opportunistic infections occur during seroconversion
    d. It is a lentivirus

18. **The following are live vaccines**
    a. Measles
    b. Hepatitis B
    c. BCG
    d. Influenza

19. **Food poisoning**
    a. This is a notifiable disease
    b. When caused by *Staph. aureus*, it occurs 12–48 hours after ingestion of contaminated food
    c. That caused by *Shigella* spp. is associated with acute, watery, bloody diarrhoea
    d. *Salmonella* food poisoning is most likely if accompanied by severe abdominal pain

20. **Osteomyelitis in children**
    a. This results mostly from staphylococcal infection
    b. When caused by *Haemophilus* sp., it occurs as a complication of sickle cell disease
    c. It most commonly arises from overlying trauma
    d. It most commonly affects the femur

21. **B lymphocytes**
    a. These are produced in the bone marrow before maturing in thymic tissue
    b. They are the predominant circulating lymphocytes
    c. The primary function is antibody production
    d. They act as antigen-presenting cells

22. **The following virus and method of spread associations are correct**
    a. Adenovirus – faecal–oral
    b. Varicella – airborne
    c. CMV – blood borne
    d. Hepatitis A – blood borne

23. **Defects in the immune response and associated pathogens are as follows**
    a. Complement deficiency – *Candida* spp.
    b. Complement deficiency – *Neisseria* spp.
    c. T-cell deficiency – CMV
    d. Neutropenia – *Candida* spp.

24. **Tetanus**
    a. *Cl. tetani* is a facultative anaerobic bacillus
    b. The neurotoxin tetanospasmin blocks acetylcholine transmission
    c. Tetanospasmin reversibly binds to peripheral nerve terminals
    d. Recovery from tetanus does not confer immunity

25. **The following antiviral drug and viral pathogen pairings are correct**
    a. Ribavirin – influenza
    b. Amantadine – influenza
    c. Aciclovir – CMV
    d. Oseltamivir – RSV

1a. F
1b. F
1c. F
1d. T
Neisseria meningitidis, an encapsulated Gram-negative diplococcus, is found as part of the normal oral flora in up to 40% of healthy young adults. Transmission is by droplet or direct contact. Vaccines are available for meningitis A, C, Y and W135, but not for meningitis B.

2a. F
2b. F
2c. F
2d. T
HSV (herpes simplex virus) encephalitis predominantly affects the temporal lobes. The usual clinical course is fever, headache and confusion over several days, often accompanied by altered behaviour and hallucinations. It is a serious life-threatening condition causing cerebral oedema and a severe haemorrhagic, necrotising encephalitis. The mortality rate is 70% if untreated and 19% when treated with aciclovir. It is diagnosed by PCR (polymerase chain reaction) on CSF (cerebrospinal fluid) with a test sensitivity of 99%.

3a. F
3b. T
3c. T
3d. F
Transplacental transfer of maternally generated antibodies (IgG) provides newborn immunity. IgM is the major antibody of the primary immune response and its presence indicates recent infection. Splenectomy predisposes to infection with encapsulated bacteria such as *Streptococcus*, *Haemophilus* and *Neisseria* spp. Cryptococcal infections occur in conditions of reduced T-cell-mediated immunity (AIDS, Hodgkin's lymphoma, corticosteroid therapy).

4a. F
4b. T
4c. T
4d. F
UK notifiable diseases (to the consultant in Communicable Disease Control) are:

- Anthrax
- Cholera
- Diphtheria
- Dysentery
- Encephalitis
- Food poisoning
- Leprosy

- Leptospirosis
- Malaria
- Measles
- Meningitis
- Meningococcal sepsis
- Mumps
- Ophthalmia neonatorum
- Pertussis
- Plague
- Polio
- Rabies
- Relapsing fever
- Rubella
- Scarlet fever
- Tetanus
- Tuberculosis
- Typhus
- Viral haemorrhagic fever
- Viral hepatitis

Reporting of HIV infection is voluntary and anonymous.

5a. F
5b. F
5c. T
5d. T
Only 5% of neutrophils are in the peripheral circulating pool, 85% are in bone marrow and the remaining 10% are adherent to endothelial surfaces. Integrins mediate adhesion and opsonin (specific antibodies and complement) binds to antigens to facilitate phagocytosis. A transient rise in neutrophil counts occurs after exercise due to movement of the marginal pool (endothelial neutrophils) into the circulation. This also occurs after a seizure and a tachycardia.

6a. F
6b. T
6c. F
6d. F
Sputum culture in miliary TB is negative in 80% of cases; the spread is haematogenous. Up to 50% of cases are diagnosed only post-mortem. As the bacterium is haematogenous rather than endobronchial, it is not as contagious as pulmonary TB. The CSF in tuberculous meningitis shows elevated protein levels and low glucose levels.

7a. T
7b. F
7c. F
7d. F
Toxic shock syndrome results from staphylococci that produce the exotoxin TSST-1, which non-specifically binds to the major histocompatibility complex and T cells, resulting in polyclonal T-cell activation. Half of cases

are menstrually related, the remainder occurring in men/children associated with breaches to the skin. Classically the rash is a 'sunburn'-like diffuse macular erythema.

8a. F
8b. F
8c. T
8d. F
Clostridia are spore-forming Gram-positive, anaerobic bacilli and are ubiquitous in the environment. Pathogenic species include *Cl. perfringens*, *Cl. tetani*, *Cl. difficile* and *Cl. botulinum*. *Cl. perfringens* releases exotoxins that cause tissue necrosis in gas gangrene or diarrhoea in food poisoning.

Cl. difficile causes antibiotic-associated diarrhoea, colitis and pseudomembranous colitis. It occurs following disturbance of the normal gastrointestinal (GI) tract flora post-antibiotic use, but may also occur in immunocompromised individuals or after GI surgery.

9a. F
9b. F
9c. T
9d. T
Malaria is caused by *Plasmodium* spp. and transmitted by the female *Anopheles* mosquito. *P. falciparum* causes the most severe, life-threatening form of the disease and *P. vivax* is the commonest cause of benign malaria. *P. vivax* and *P. ovale* have dormant liver stage parasites (hypnozoites) that may relapse months or years after the infecting bite. *P. malariae* can persist asymptomatically for many years. Serial blood films are required to exclude malaria.

10a. F
10b. T
10c. F
10d. F
The UK immunisation schedule is as follows:

Age	Vaccinations
2 months	Diphtheria, tetanus, pertussis, polio and *Haemophilus influenzae* type b (DTaP/IPV/Hib), pneumococcal (PCV)
3 months	DTaP/IPV/Hib, meningitis C (Men C)
4 months	DTaP/IPV/Hib, PCV, Men C
12 months	Hib/Men C
13 months	MMR, PCV
3 years 4 months	DTaP/IPV or DTaP/IPV, MMR
13–18 years	Td/IPV

Vaccine against chickenpox is generally only given to non-immune children with a high-risk sibling, e.g. leukaemia, or non-immune healthcare workers. Measles, mumps and rubella (MMR) and BCG (bacille Calmette–Guérin) are live, attenuated vaccines. Tetanus and diphtheria are toxoids.

11a. F
11b. T
11c. F
11d. F

Weil's disease is caused by *Leptospira interrogans*. *Borrelia burgdorferi*, another spirochaete, causes Lyme disease. A rhabdovirus is the cause of rabies. Dengue, a viral haemorrhagic fever, is the most prevalent arbovirus disease. A rotavirus causes gastroenteritis. Bronchiolitis is commonly due to RSV (respiratory syncytial virus) infection.

12a. F
12b. T
12c. F
12d. F

PID usually results from ascending genital tract infection. Over half is caused by chlamydial infection, gonorrhoea accounting for up to 20%. Chlamydial infection may be associated with a perihepatitis (Curtis−Fitz−Hugh syndrome), causing right upper quadrant pain.

Antibiotic treatment of acute PID should be commenced early to reduce the complications, e.g. tubal infertility.

13a. F
13b. F
13c. F
13d. T

The most common infective cause of bacterial endocarditis is *Strep. viridans*. Staphylococcal endocarditis is most commonly seen in normal native valve endocarditis and in intravenous drug users. Infection with *Strep. bovis* is associated with underlying gastrointestinal pathology/malignancy.
Several separate blood cultures may be required to confirm the causative organism, particularly in Gram-negative infections on native valves with the slow-growing HACEK group of organisms (*Haemophilus, Actinobacillus, Cardiobacterium, Eikenella* and *Kingella* spp.). Culture-negative endocarditis is seen with *Coxiella burnettii, Chlamydia psittaci*, fastidious streptococci, mycobacteria and fungi (*Aspergillus* spp.).

14a. T
14b. T
14c. F
14d. F

Myocarditis with an infective aetiology is seen with viral (HIV, Coxsackievirus, enterovirus, rubella, polio, cytomegalovirus or CMV), bacterial (*Brucella* and *Corynebacterium* spp., and gonoccoci) and spirochaetal (*Borrelia* spp., leptospirosis) diseases. Worldwide the most common cause is the trypanosomal Chagas' disease.

Strep. viridans is the leading cause of endocarditis.

15a. T
15b. F
15c. F
15d. T
Viral meningitis is very common and usually mild, the importance lying in differentiating it from more serious bacterial/mycobacterial meningitis. The CSF in viral meningitis typically shows a lymphocytosis, raised protein and slightly lowered glucose.

Viral meningitis most commonly occurs in children and is due to enterovirus infection (echovirus, Coxsackievirus, mumps) occurring in epidemics, usually in late summer. Herpes simplex virus (HSV) type 1 causes encephalitis and type 2 occasionally causes meningitis.

16a. T
16b. F
16c. T
16d. F
Streptococcal virulence is enhanced by producing streptokinase (lyses blood clots, facilitating spread), streptolysin (lyses leukocytes, platelets and erythrocytes), pyrogenic exotoxins, DNAase and peptidase.

F-proteins enhance adhesion to epithelial cells. M-proteins aid adhesion, act as antiphagocytotics and degrade complement (cross-reactivity leads to rheumatic fever). Phagocytosis is inhibited by the presence of a cellular capsule.

Panton–Valentine leukocidin is a potent neutrophil-lysing cytotoxin produced by *Staph. aureus*.

17a. F
17b. F
17c. T
17d. T
In the UK (as opposed to the USA) the diagnosis of AIDS is based on the presence of specific indicator diseases, not absolute CD4 counts. HIV is a lentivirus. After infection seroconversion usually occurs between 6 and 8 weeks (range 4–12). It is associated with a high viral load and profound fall in CD4 count, which may predispose to opportunistic pneumocystis or *Candida* infection.

18a. T
18b. F
18c. T
18d. F
Measles, mumps, rubella, Sabin oral polio, yellow fever, BCG and typhoid are live attenuated vaccines. Hepatitis B is a recombinant vaccine and influenza is an inactivated conjugate vaccine.

19a. T
19b. F
19c. T
19d. F
Food poisoning caused by *Staph. aureus* occurs rapidly, 2–4 hours after
ingestion of a pre-formed toxin. Bloody diarrhoea (dysentery) is seen with
Shigella and *Campylobacter* spp. *Salmonella* sp. has an incubation of 12–36
hours with vomiting and fever followed by watery-brown to green diarrhoea.
It is one of the most common causes of persisting diarrhoea without
abdominal pain.

20a. T
20b. F
20c. F
20d. T
Over 90% of childhood osteomyelitis is caused by staphylococci. *Salmonella* sp.
complicates sickle cell disease. Osteomyelitis most commonly arises by
haematogenous spread to the metaphysis of the long bones (35% femur,
30% tibia).

21a. F
21b. F
21c. T
21d. T
B lymphocytes are produced in the bone marrow and mature in the bursa
equivalent, including marrow and Peyer's patch, fetal liver and spleen. Primarily
acting to produce antibodies, B lymphocytes also act to present antigen to T
cells, which constitute 60–80% of peripheral lymphocytes.

22a. T
22b. T
22c. T
22d. F
Adenovirus is transmitted via aerosol, close contact and faecal–oral routes.
Airborne virus transmission occurs with varicella, paramyxovirus, influenza,
rhinovirus, enterovirus and parvovirus. Blood-borne transmission occurs with
HIV, hepatitis B, C and D, and CMV. Hepatitis A is faecal–oral. Transmission by
direct contact occurs with herpes simplex, EBV (Epstein–Barr virus), CMV
and poxvirus.

23a. F
23b. T
23c. T
23d. T
Complement deficiency predisposes to infections with staphylococci,
streptococci, and *Proteus*, *Pseudomonas* and *Neisseria* spp. B-cell deficiency
predisposes the individual to infection with enterovirus, staphylococci,
streptococci, *Haemophilus*, *Neisseria* and *Pneumocystis* spp., and *E. coli*. A lack of
T-cell function is associated with infections with CMV, HSV, HZV (herpes

zoster virus), *Listeria* sp., mycobacteria, cryptococci, and *Nocardia, Aspergillus, Candida, Histoplasma* and *Pneumocystis* spp.

24a. F
24b. F
24c. F
24d. T

Clostridium tetani is a strictly anaerobic, spore-forming bacillus which dies rapidly on exposure to oxygen. The toxin produced, tetanospasmin, irreversibly binds to axonal terminals, blocking the release of GABA (γ-aminobutyric acid) at the inhibitory synapse. Unregulated excitatory activation causes the spastic paralysis seen in tetanus. Botulinum toxin blocks acetylcholine transmission.

25a. F
25b. T
25c. F
25d. F

Aciclovir and famciclovir are active against HSV and zaricella-zoster. CMV is treated with ganciclovir or foscarnet. Amantadine, oseltamivir and zanamivir are used to treat influenza. Ribavirin is used to treat RSV, Lassa fever and hepatitis C.

5. Clinical conundrums: Questions

1. Thyrotoxic crisis
a. This is a laboratory diagnosis
b. It is associated with hyperglycaemia
c. Aspirin should be avoided
d. It causes an elevated serum calcium

2. Bacterial meningitis
a. In neonates it is most commonly caused by β-haemolytic streptococci
b. It is now preventable as a result of the introduction of the meningococcal vaccine
c. That caused by pneumococci has an identical rash to meningococcal disease
d. That caused by tuberculosis is more common in adults

3. Basal skull fracture should be suspected in the presence of the following
a. Subhyaloid haemorrhage
b. Anosmia
c. Fluid level in the maxillary sinus
d. Bruising over the mastoid process

4. In trauma patients
a. Bradycardia and hypotension suggest spinal shock
b. Bradycardia and hypertension suggest raised intracranial pressure
c. A 750 mL blood loss will result in decreased urine output
d. A normal blood pressure excludes significant blood loss

5. Regarding shoulder dislocations
a. Posterior dislocations are the most common
b. They are associated with damage to the musculocutaneous nerve
c. They are rare in children
d. The lesser tuberosity is often displaced

6. Hyponatraemia
a. Rapid correction of the sodium level should be avoided to prevent subacute combined cord degeneration
b. Addison's disease may be the cause
c. It may follow Ecstasy ingestion in young adults
d. A urinary sodium of 30 mmol/L will be seen in hypovolaemic hyponatraemia

7. **Horner's syndrome**
   a. This results from interruption to the parasympathetic supply to the eye
   b. It is associated with miosis
   c. It is associated with decreased eye abduction
   d. It is associated with ptosis

8. **Sickle cell anaemia**
   a. This may present with priapism
   b. Aplastic crises are commonly precipitated by parvovirus infections
   c. It is associated with an increased susceptibility to gallstones
   d. Vasoocclusive crises are associated with a drop in haemoglobin

9. **In acute pancreatitis**
   a. Hypoglycaemia is a marker of increased severity
   b. An amylase rise of less than four times normal indicates mild disease
   c. The most common cause is gallstones
   d. It may result from bike 'handlebar' injuries

10. **In patients presenting to the emergency department (ED) after an overdose**
    a. N-Acetylcysteine should be administered as early as possible in paracetamol poisoning
    b. Naloxone has a short half-life
    c. A trial of flumazenil is recommended in suspected benzodiazepine overdose
    d. Tricyclic antidepressant overdose is associated with prolongation of P–R interval on the ECG

11. **In acute stroke**
    a. Middle cerebral artery (MCA) territory strokes may lead to contralateral hemiplegia
    b. Primary intracerebral haemorrhage accounts for 25% of cases
    c. Brain-stem strokes may result in deafness
    d. Early neurosurgical intervention is useful in anterior artery territory stroke

12. **Hydrostatic pulmonary oedema is seen in the following**
    a. Left ventricular failure
    b. ARDS
    c. Pulmonary emboli
    d. Liver failure

13. **The following are all components of the systemic inflammatory response syndrome (SIRS)**
    a. A temperature of <36 °C
    b. A systolic blood pressure <90 mmHg
    c. A heart rate >90 beats/min
    d. Oxygen saturations of <92% on air

14. **The following are tetanus-prone wounds**
    a. Wound >6 hours old
    b. A burn with a significant degree of devitalised tissue
    c. Heavy contamination, especially with soil or faeces
    d. Puncture wounds

15. **In patients with a suspected ectopic pregnancy**
    a. A negative urine β human chorionic gonadotrophin (βhCG) safely rules out pregnancy
    b. A high serum βhCG confirms that a pregnancy is intrauterine
    c. They may present with shoulder tip pain
    d. Transvaginal ultrasonography may be better than transabdominal ultrasonography

16. **Patients who have had a TIA**
    a. The risk of subsequent stroke increases if the patient has diabetes and the symptoms lasted more than 2 hours
    b. They should never be given aspirin because this may cause bleeding
    c. Most patients do not require follow-up and can be discharged
    d. The TIA may be associated with temporal arteritis or SLE

17. **In patients with headache**
    a. The presence of jaw claudication suggests trigeminal neuralgia
    b. Cluster headaches are more common in males
    c. Temporal arteritis usually causes a rise in the erythrocyte sedimentation rate
    d. Risk factors associated with central venous thrombosis include use of the oral contraceptive pill and malignancy

18. **A prolonged Q–T interval on an ECG may be caused by the following**
    a. Hypomagnesaemia
    b. Hyperkalaemia
    c. Raised intracranial pressure
    d. Hypothermia

19. Pain in the malleolar zone and which of the following criteria form part of the Ottawa ankle rule
    a. Bone tenderness along the distal 6 cm of the posterior edge of the tibia or tip of the medial malleolus
    b. Bone tenderness at the base of the fifth metatarsal
    c. An inability to bear weight both immediately and in the ED for four steps
    d. Bone tenderness along the distal 6 cm of the posterior edge of the fibula or tip of the lateral malleolus

20. Causes of a raised anion gap acidosis include the following
    a. Methanol ingestion
    b. Renal tubular acidosis
    c. Carbon monoxide poisoning
    d. Diarrhoea

21. According to the NICE guidelines, adult patients with which of the following should be considered for immediate CT of the brain after head injury
    a. Age >65 years
    b. Focal neurological deficit
    c. GCS <15
    d. Seizures

22. The incubation period of the following infections is less than 1 week
    a. Chickenpox
    b. Meningococci
    c. Epstein–Barr virus
    d. Gonorrhoea

23. Hormonal emergency contraception
    a. It is more effective than the insertion of an intrauterine device
    b. It is effective if taken within 4 days of unprotected intercourse
    c. The efficacy decreases the longer the delay between unprotected intercourse and taking it
    d. If vomiting occurs within 2 hours of taking it, another dose should be taken

24. During pregnancy the following physiological changes occur
    a. An increase in peripheral vascular resistance
    b. A decrease in diastolic blood pressure
    c. An increase in cardiac output
    d. An increase in blood volume and haemoglobin concentration

25. The following are poor prognostic indicators after drowning
    a. Hypothermia
    b. Immersion for more than 5 min
    c. Teenagers
    d. Saltwater immersion

5. Clinical conundrums: Answers

1a. F
1b. F
1c. T
1d. T

Thyrotoxicosis is a clinical diagnosis. Thyroid function tests (TFTs) provide no discrimination between thyrotoxicosis and crisis. The hypercatabolic state rapidly depletes hepatic glycogen stores, resulting in hypoglycaemia. Salicylates displace thyroxine (T_4) from thyroid-binding globulin (TBG), worsening the thyroid storm.

2a. T
2b. F
2c. F
2d. F

Bacterial meningitis in neonates is most frequently caused by β-haemolytic streptococci and *Escherichia coli* infection. Most cases result from meningococcal infection. Immunisation is against meningococcal C but most disease is the result of meningococcal B. Pneumococcal disease is the second most common cause of bacterial meningitis in the UK. It is usually not associated with septicaemia and a rash is very rarely seen. Tuberculous meningitis is more common in young children.

3a. F
3b. T
3c. F
3d. T

Clinical signs of basal skull fracture include subconjunctival haemorrhages, bruising over the mastoid processes (Battle's sign), periorbital bruising (panda eyes), haemotympanum, CSF (cerebrospinal fluid) or blood otorrhoea or rhinorrhoea. Anosmia may result from tearing of olfactory fibres as they pass through the cribriform plate. Subhyaloid haemorrhages are small vitreous haemorrhages.

4a. F
4b. T
4c. F
4d. F

Neurogenic shock should be suspected in the presence of bradycardia and hypotension, together with vasodilatation. Spinal shock is the sensory loss and paralysis associated with spinal cord injury. According to ATLS (Advanced Trauma Life Support) principles, a blood loss of 750 mL (category I shock) results in tachycardia. Blood pressure (BP) is maintained until late, especially in young fit adults. The systolic BP falls and urinary output falls only once approximately 30% of the blood volume (1500 mL) has been lost.

5a. F
5b. T
5c. T
5d. F
Anterior dislocations are by far the most common shoulder dislocation. They are seen most often in young adults and elderly people but rarely in children. The most common neurological complication seen is axillary nerve palsy: loss of sensation over 'regimental badge' area and weak abduction. Musculocutaneous nerve injury can occur, causing loss sensation on the radial side of the forearm and weakness of supination and elbow flexion. Anterior dislocations result in damage to the capsule and displacement of the glenoid labrum (Bankart's lesion).

6a. F
6b. T
6c. T
6d. F
Rapid correction of low sodium levels may result in central pontine myelinolysis. Chronic hyponatraemia should be corrected slowly (maximum 0.5 mmol/L per h up to 120 mmol/L). Acute symptomatic hyponatraemia can be corrected at 2 mmol/L per h at most. Mineralocorticoid deficiency results in hyponatraemia and hyperkalaemia. Hyponatraemia can be classified depending on the fluid status, normovolaemic hyponatraemia (SIADH [syndrome of inappropriate antidiuretic hormone secretion], postoperative inappropriate dextrose infusion), hypovolaemic hyponatraemia (D&V [diarrhoea and vomiting], burns, excessive prolonged sweating) and hypervolaemic hyponatraemia (cardiac failure, cirrhosis, nephrotic syndrome). Hyponatraemia after Ecstasy ingestion is seen as a result of excessive sweating; consumption of large volumes of water contributes.

7a. F
7b. T
7c. F
7d. T
Horner's syndrome is caused by interruption of the sympathetic chain. It results in miosis, ptosis, enophthalmus and decreased sweating to the ipsilateral side. A lateral rectus palsy (nerve VI) causes failure/weakness of eye abduction.

8a. T
8b. T
8c. T
8d. F
Sickle cell anaemia, an autosomal recessive disorder, is associated with an increased susceptibility to gallstones, meningitis, osteomyelitis and avascular necrosis. Haemoglobin levels may normally be 6–8 g/dL but fall in aplastic crisis, haemolytic crisis and sequestration. Vasoocclusive crises cause pain from infarction in the liver, spleen or bone, or priapism.

9a. F
9b. F
9c. T
9d. T

In acute pancreatitis, amylase levels are not an indicator of severity. Markers of severity at presentation include age >55, white cell count >16, glucose >10, LDH (lactate dehydrogenase) >350 and AST (aspartate transaminase) >250.

Gallstones are the most common aetiology in pancreatitis with alcohol ingestion the second. Rarer causes include iatrogenic, trauma, hypothermia and infection with mumps, rubella, Coxsackievirus or EBV (Epstein–Barr virus).

10a. F
10b. T
10c. F
10d. F

N-Acetylcysteine should be administered within 8 hours of paracetamol overdose to have maximum benefit. It should be given if only paracetamol levels are known, unless more than 8 hours have elapsed after ingestion, because adverse reactions are common, particularly if paracetamol levels are low. Naloxone has a half-life of about 1 hour, less than most opiates. Flumazenil should be used only to reverse benzodiazepines in anaesthetic/sedation procedures. Given in overdoses it may induce seizures, particularly in mixed overdoses including tricyclic antidepressants (TCAs). ECG changes associated with TCA overdoses are caused by Na^+ channel blockade and include QRS prolongation (>100 ms is significant poisoning; >160 ms precedes the development of arrhythmias).

11a. T
11b. F
11c. T
11d. F

MCA territory strokes result in contralateral hemiplegia, hemiparaesthesia and homonymous hemianopia. Primary haemorrhagic strokes account for about 15%; approximately 80% are thromboembolic in origin. Brain-stem CVAs (cerebrovascular accidents), via damage to either the cranial nerve VIII nucleus or the fascicle, may result in deafness. Cerebellar strokes, because of mass effects in the posterior fossa, may require urgent surgical decompression.

12a. T
12b. F
12c. T
12d. F

Pulmonary oedema results from a number of mechanisms:

- Hydrostatic: as occurs with raised pulmonary vasculature pressures as in left ventricular failure and PE (pulmonary embolism)
- Increased permeability as in ARDS (acute respiratory distress syndrome)

- Decreased alveolar interstitial pressures as seen in airway obstruction
- Failure of lymphatic clearance
- Hypoproteinaemic states such as liver failure where there is a decreased plasma colloid osmotic pressure.

13a. T
13b. F
13c. T
13d. F
The SIRS is evidence of a system-wide inflammatory process. It is most often used to describe a patient with sepsis who has two or more SIRS criteria and a source of infection. It can also be present with other conditions common in the ED such as trauma, PE, MI (myocardial infarction) and anaphylaxis. For a patient to be described as having SIRS he or she must have two or more of the following criteria:

- Temperature <36 °C or >38 °C
- White cell count $<4\times10^9$ or $>12\times10^9$ or >10% band forms
- Respiratory rate <20 breaths/min or $PaCO_2$ <4.3 kPa (32 mmHg)
- Heart rate >90 beats/min.

14a. T
14b. T
14c. T
14d. T
The need for administration of tetanus vaccine or immunoglobulin after injury depends on a patient's immunisation status and whether the wound is 'tetanus prone'. Individuals are considered to have life-long immunity if they received a full course of five tetanus vaccinations in early life. There is no longer a need for individuals to receive immunisation every 10 years. A wound is considered tetanus prone if there is:

- Heavy contamination (especially with soil of faeces)
- Devitalised tissue
- Wounds >6 hours old
- Puncture wounds and animal bites.

15a. F
15b. F
15c. T
15d. T
The frequency of ectopic pregnancy (implantation of the gestational sac outside the uterus) has increased over recent years and now occurs in about 1 in 100 pregnancies. A urine βhCG is almost always positive but may be negative. A high serum βhCG does not confirm that the pregnancy is intrauterine. The classic presentation of a patient with ectopic pregnancy is unilateral severe abdominal pain, collapse and vaginal bleeding. Patients may present with shoulder tip pain caused by intraperitoneal fluid irritating the diaphragm.

16a. T
16b. F
16c. F
16d. T
A transient ischaemic attack (TIA) is defined as an episode of focal neurological deficit that lasts less than 24 hours (although most resolve within 2 hours). Many patients who have a TIA will go on to have a stroke, and all patients who present with symptoms of a TIA should be observed to ensure that symptoms resolve and that suitable follow-up is arranged. All patients should be started on aspirin unless there is a compelling reason not to. TIAs are associated with hypertension, sickle cell disease, vasculitis (such as temporal arteritis or systemic lupus erythematosus [SLE]) and syphilis. To try to estimate a subsequent risk of stroke the ABCD2 score can be used.

17a. F
17b. T
17c. T
17d. T
Headache is a common presentation to the ED. There are several serious causes of headache that must be actively excluded. Temporal (or giant cell) arteritis occurs more often in patients over the age of 50 and may present with visual disturbance or jaw claudication. It usually causes a rise in the ESR. Cluster headaches occur more commonly in males (about 90%), often at night, and may respond to high-flow oxygen therapy. Risk factors associated with central venous thrombosis include use of the oral contraceptive pill, pregnancy and the puerperium, dehydration, haematological disorders such as polycythaemia, malignancy and direct spread of infection from neighbouring sites.

18a. T
18b. F
18c. T
18d. T
A prolonged Q–T interval on an ECG is important to recognise because it may be a cause of torsades de pointes, ventricular fibrillation and sudden death. Causes of a prolonged Q–T interval include hypokalaemia, hypomagnesaemia, hypocalcaemia, hypothermia, acute MI, drugs that block sodium channels, raised intracranial pressure and congenital disorders.

19a. T
19b. F
19c. T
19d. T
The Ottawa ankle rule was introduced after large-scale derivation and validation studies to try to reduce the number of unnecessary ankle radiographs being performed in the ED. There are also rules for foot and knee radiographs.

The Ottawa ankle rule states that patients need a series of ankle radiographs only if they have pain in the malleolar zone and any of the following:

- Bone tenderness along the distal 6 cm of the posterior edge of the tibia or tip of the medial malleolus

- Bone tenderness along the distal 6 cm of the posterior edge of the fibula or tip of the lateral malleolus
- An inability to bear weight both immediately and in the ED for four steps.

Pain at the base of the fifth metatarsal is part of the Ottawa foot rule.

20a. T
20b. F
20c. T
20d. F
The anion gap is calculated using the formula $(Na^+ + K^+) - (HCO_3^- + Cl^-)$ and usually lies between 14 and 18. Causes of a raised anion gap acidosis can be remembered using the mnemonic CAT MUD PILES:

Carbon monoxide or **C**yanide poisoning
Alcohol
Toluene
Methanol
Uraemia
Diabetic ketoacidosis
Paraldehyde
Isoniazid
Lactic acidosis
Ethylene glycol
Salicylates

Diarrhoea and renal tubular acidosis cause a normal anion gap acidosis.

21a. F
21b. T
21c. F
21d. T
The NICE (National Institute for Health and Clinical Excellence) head injury guidelines suggest performing an immediate CT brain scan in adult patients with any of the following:

- GCS (Glasgow Coma Scale) <13 on initial assessment in the ED
- GCS <15 when assessed in the ED 2 hours after injury
- Suspected open or depressed skull fracture
- Any sign of basal skull fracture (haemotympanum, 'panda' eyes, CSF leakage from the ear or nose, Battle's sign)
- Post-traumatic seizure
- Focal neurological deficit
- More than one episode of vomiting
- Amnesia for events more than 30 min before impact
- Patients who have experienced some loss of consciousness before the injury and:
  - age 65 years or older
  - coagulopathy (history of bleeding, clotting disorder, current treatment with warfarin)

– dangerous mechanism of injury (a pedestrian or cyclist struck by a motor vehicle, an occupant ejected from a motor vehicle, or a fall from a height of greater than 1 metre or five stairs).

22a. F
22b. T
22c. F
22d. T
Knowledge of the incubation periods of common infectious diseases is essential when assessing patients in the ED. Approximate incubation periods of common or serious infectious disease are given below.

Incubation period

<1 week	Between 1 week and 3 weeks	>3 weeks
Meningococci	Chickenpox	HIV
Diphtheria	Measles	Hepatitis A
Gonorrhoea	Mumps	Hepatitis B
Salmonella	Rubella	Hepatitis C
	Malaria	Syphilis
	Polio	EBV
	Tetanus	
	Typhoid	

23a. F
23b. F
23c. T
23d. T
Although largely seen as the job of primary care or pharmacies, patients may still present to the ED requesting emergency contraception. Hormonal emergency contraception involves the use of levonorgestrel, which is most effective if given within 72 hours. It can be taken outside this window, but its efficacy decreases with time and use in this circumstance is unlicensed.

24a. F
24b. T
24c. T
24d. F
Certain physiological changes occur throughout pregnancy. These include:

• Increased cardiac output and blood volume
• Decreased peripheral vascular resistance
• Decreased blood pressure (especially diastolic)
• Decreased haemoglobin concentration (caused by dilution).

25a. F
25b. T
25c. F
25d. F
Although complete recovery is possible after a long period of immersion (especially if associated with hypothermia), immersion for more than 5 min is a poor prognostic sign. Patients at extremes of age are at increased risk. The type of water makes no difference to the outcome.

6. Biochemistry: Questions

1. **After an episode of trauma, the following metabolic changes occur in the human stress response**
   a. Human metabolic changes occur that inhibit a catabolic state
   b. ACTH output from the anterior pituitary gland is inhibited
   c. Vasopressin release from the posterior pituitary is increased
   d. Cortisol release from the adrenal gland is increased

2. **After an episode of trauma, the following metabolic changes occur in the human stress response**
   a. The overall effect is to mobilise substrate as an energy source
   b. Urine output is decreased
   c. Cortisol promotes gluconeogenesis in the liver
   d. Glucose uptake into cells is inhibited

3. **After an episode of trauma, the following metabolic changes occur in the human stress response**
   a. Growth hormone secretion is decreased
   b. Blood glucose levels are likely to increase
   c. Skeletal muscle cells are broken down to release amino acids
   d. Lipolysis is decreased

4. **After an episode of trauma, the following metabolic changes occur in the human stress response**
   a. Fever may be present and not indicate infection
   b. The CRP may be elevated
   c. There is a relative state of insulin resistance
   d. A D-dimer test may be elevated

5. **In glycolysis**
   a. Glucose is split to form pyruvate in all cells of the body
   b. A total of eight molecules of ATP are produced, for use by the mitochondria, when glucose is metabolised aerobically
   c. Lactate is produced when glucose is metabolised anaerobically
   d. Three ATP molecules are produced, together with two molecules of pyruvate, from glycolysis of one molecule of glucose

6. **Concerning gluconeogenesis**
   a. This process takes place mainly in skeletal muscle
   b. It is essentially the opposite of glycolysis
   c. Glucose is most commonly formed using lactate as a substrate
   d. This metabolic pathway is inhibited by insulin

7. **Sugars**
   a. Glucose is a polysaccharide
   b. Maltose is made from two units of glucose
   c. Fructose is a disaccharide
   d. Sucrose is a disaccharide made of glucose and galactose

8. **Glucagon**
   a. Glucagon induces hypoglycaemia
   b. Glucagon stimulates the release of free fatty acids from triglycerides
   c. Glucagon is produced in the β cells of the pancreatic islets of Langerhans
   d. It is initially secreted as pro-glucagon

9. **In a state of starvation, the following statements are correct:**
   a. Glucagon levels are elevated
   b. Blood sugar levels are maintained initially by breakdown of triglycerides
   c. Protein may be broken down to maintain energy levels
   d. The brain will start to utilise ketone bodies as fuel

10. **The following results are given for a patient in the emergency department (ED)**

pH	7.28
PaO_2	42.5 kPa (319 mmHg)
$PaCO_2$	2.5 kPa (18.7 mmHg)
HCO_3^-	10.0 mmol/L
BE (base excess)	−8.0
Lactate	3.7 mmol/L

    a. The patient has a respiratory acidosis
    b. The patient is likely to be tachypnoeic
    c. The chloride is likely to be normal
    d. This could be an overcompensated respiratory alkalosis

11. **The following results are given for a patient in the ED**

pH	7.58
PaO_2	15.0 kPa (112 mmHg)
$PaCO_2$	4.5 kPa (33.7 mmHg)
HCO_3^-	32.0 mmol/L
BE	+4.0
Lactate	1.7 mmol/L

    a. The patient has a metabolic alkalosis
    b. The patient may be taking diuretics
    c. The chloride is likely to be normal
    d. This could be the result of poisoning

12. **The following results are given for a patient in the ED**

    pH   7.56
    PaO_2 12.0 kPa (90 mmHg)
    $PaCO_2$ 2.5 kPa (18.8 mmHg)
    HCO_3^- 22.0 mmol/L
    BE   +4.0
    Lactate   1.4 mmol/L

    a. The patient has a metabolic alkalosis
    b. The patient may be experiencing anxiety
    c. There is no evidence of acid–base compensation
    d. The patient may be experiencing tingling in the hands and feet

13. **After alcohol intoxication, which of the following metabolic changes occur?**
    a. Hyperglycaemia
    b. An increase in uric acid production
    c. Reduced serum lactate
    d. Mild acidosis

14. **Lactate**
    a. Lactic acidosis occurs during anaerobic metabolism in muscle
    b. The serum lactate, when measured in the acute setting of trauma, has a prognostic significance
    c. The lactate level is elevated after a seizure
    d. In the setting of sepsis, an initial lactate of 2.5 mmol/L indicates septic shock

15. **The hypothalamic–pituitary–thyroid axis**
    a. Thyroid-stimulating hormone (TSH) is produced by the posterior pituitary
    b. The hypothalamus produces thyrotrophin-releasing hormone (TRH), which inhibits release of TSH
    c. T_3 and T_4 are both produced in equal amounts by the thyroid gland
    d. T_3 and T_4 are mostly inactive and bound to thyroxine-binding globulin (TBG)

16. **Parathyroid hormone**
    a. This increases osteoclastic activity in bone
    b. Secretion results in a high serum calcium and a high serum phosphate
    c. Levels are increased in patients with multiple endocrine neoplasia
    d. Secretion reduces vitamin D production

17. **Cortisol**
    a. This is secreted from the zona glomerulosa of the adrenal cortex
    b. It is secreted in a diurnal rhythm, with secretion being highest at night
    c. Secretion results in stimulation of lipolysis
    d. It has a role in the formation of short-term emotional memories

18. **Cushing's disease**
    a. The usual cause is adrenal hyperplasia
    b. ACTH levels are usually high
    c. Excess cortisol will be secreted in the urine
    d. A raised 24-hour urine 5-hydroxyindoleacetic acid (5-HIAA) level is diagnostic

19. **Addison's disease**
    a. Patients often present with hyponatraemia
    b. There is a positive association in patients with HIV/AIDS
    c. It may be associated with Graves' disease
    d. ACTH levels are often low

20. **Conn's syndrome**
    a. Patients often present with hyponatraemia
    b. A normal potassium effectively excludes the diagnosis
    c. Plasma renin levels are high
    d. Patients may present with hypertension

21. **Growth hormone**
    a. This is released in a constant fashion from the anterior pituitary gland
    b. Sleep acts to stimulate its release
    c. Glucose acts to inhibit its release
    d. It is generally a catabolic substance

22. **Renin–angiotensin system**
    a. Renin is produced by the juxtaglomerular cells of the kidney
    b. Renin levels are likely to be high in a patient with a haemorrhage
    c. Renin converts angiotensin I to angiotensin II
    d. Angiotensin II will result in increased aldosterone release

23. **Thiamine deficiency is associated with which of the following?**
    a. Cardiac failure
    b. Weight loss
    c. Angular stomatitis
    d. Peripheral neuropathy

24. **Which of the following may be associated with hypoglycaemia?**
    a. Alcohol intoxication
    b. Acromegaly
    c. Hepatocellular failure
    d. Acute pancreatitis

25. Blood results on a patient in your ED show:

    - Severe elevation of alanine transaminase (ALT)
    - Mild elevation of alkaline phosphatase (ALP)
    - Mild elevation of bilirubin.

    Which of the following are possible diagnoses?
    a. Paracetamol poisoning
    b. Alcoholic cirrhosis
    c. Gallstones
    d. Acute viral hepatitis A

6. Biochemistry: Answers

1a. F
1b. F
1c. T
1d. T
During the human stress response there is increased secretion of pituitary hormones, promoting a catabolic state. Increased secretion of ACTH, vasopressin and cortisol increases the breakdown of fat, protein and glycogen, and stimulates the production of glucose.

2a. T
2b. T
2c. T
2d. T
During trauma the body's primary aim is to mobilise energy sources and retain circulating volume. Hormonal effects increase the production of glucose and retain fluid via the kidneys, as well as promoting widespread vasoconstriction to maintain circulating blood flow.

3a. F
3b. T
3c. T
3d. F
The stress response causes an increased level of growth hormone to be released. Fat, protein and glycogen are all broken down into easily utilised energy sources.

4a. T
4b. T
4c. T
4d. T
The stress response is the name given to a set of hormonal, neuroendocrine and metabolic changes that follow surgery and trauma.

Generally there is increased secretion of pituitary hormones, which promotes a state of catabolism and mobilises substrates to provide energy for the body to recover. This includes:

- Increased adrenocorticotrophin hormone (ACTH) and growth hormone (GH) secretion (promotes a catabolic state and causes insulin resistance)
- Decreased thyroxine secretion
- Increased vasopressin secretion
- Increased cortisol and aldosterone secretion
- Decreased insulin secretion
- Increased glucagon secretion

- Increased cytokine production (interleukin 6 [IL-6], tumour necrosis factor [TNF])
- Neutrophil leukocytosis
- Lymphocyte proliferation.

These all lead to a catabolic state so breakdown of fat, protein and glycogen is promoted, as is the production of glucose.

5a. T
5b. T
5c. T
5d. F
Glycolysis is the start of the body's processes to manufacture ATP using glucose. When oxygen is available, pyruvate is produced, with a total of eight molecules of ATP being formed after the reduction of NADH to $NADH_2$. Anaerobic respiration results in the formation of lactate.

6a. F
6b. T
6c. T
6d. T
Glycolysis is the splitting of glucose in the cytosol of all cells in the body. It occurs, with variations, in almost all organisms, both aerobic and anaerobic. Aerobic metabolism of one molecule of glucose will result in two molecules of ATP, two molecules of pyruvate and two molecules of NADH (each of which can produce three molecules of ATP when they are reduced to $NADH_2$). The pyruvate generated is then available for the tricarboxylic or citric acid cycle which occurs in the mitochondria. In anaerobic glycolysis there is an increased production of lactate, with a reduced yield of ATP. Intracellular regulators of this process include amino acids, the citric acid cycle intermediate citrate, and the acyl intermediates acetyl-CoA and fatty acids. All of these stimulate gluconeogenesis and inhibit glycolysis. In addition, the energy level of a cell controls glycolysis and gluconeogenesis. When energy levels are low (AMP, ADP), glycolysis is stimulated, whereas high energy levels (ATP) inhibit glycolysis and activate gluconeogenesis. Hormones are extracellular regulators that also affect glycolysis and gluconeogenesis. They coordinate metabolic activity among different organs. Insulin stimulates glycolysis to lower blood glucose levels after a meal, whereas glucagon and adrenaline (epinephrine) stimulate gluconeogenesis (and lipolysis in fatty tissue by hepatic lipase) to provide energy to muscle and brain during stress. Gluconeogenesis is essentially the opposite of glycolysis except that it occurs mainly in liver cells. The most common substrate is lactate but amino acids can also be converted to glucose, as can uneven-chain fatty acids.

7a. F
7b. T
7c. F
7d. F
The monosaccharides are glucose, galactose and fructose. The disaccharides are maltose (two glucose molecules), sucrose (glucose + fructose) and lactose (galactose + glucose).

8a. F
8b. T
8c. F
8d. T

Both insulin and glucagon, together with somatostatin, are secreted from the islets of Langerhans in the pancreas. α Cells produce glucagon and sit in the periphery of the islets together with the δ cells that produce somatostatin. The central β cells produce insulin. Both insulin and glucagon are secreted as pre-hormones. In general, insulin is anabolic and glucagon is catabolic. The effects of both are summarised below.

Insulin
Stimulates synthesis of triglycerides (TGs) from free fatty acids (FFAs) and inhibits release of FFAs from TGs. It increases synthesis of hepatic glycogen and thereby glucose uptake and storage. It inhibits hepatic gluconeogenesis, thus saving amino acids. It stimulates glucose uptake in skeletal muscle, which is then stored as glycogen and used in energy metabolism.

Insulin stimulates amino acid uptake in skeletal muscle and is essential for protein synthesis; it also reduces hunger by a hypothalamic effect on the brain.

Glucagon
Glucagon stimulates release of FFAs from TGs. It stimulates glycogenolysis and glucose release and gluconeogenesis.

9a. T
9b. F
9c. T
9d. T

In a starved state insulin levels will be low and glucagon levels high, promoting a catabolic state. Initially gluconeogenesis and glycogenolysis are upregulated in the liver. The TGs in adipose tissue are converted to fatty acids and glycerol (lipolysis), and then protein is broken down to mobilise energy. In prolonged starvation brain tissue will utilise ketone bodies from the liver as energy.

10a. F
10b. T
10c. T
10d. F

When looking at blood gas results, first look at the pH (normal range 7.35–7.45).

• Do you have an acidosis or an alkalosis?

Then look at the CO_2 (an acidic gas):

• Is this in keeping with the pH?

If you have an acidosis and the CO_2 is high (in keeping), this must be a primary respiratory acidosis.

If you have an alkalosis and the CO_2 is high, this must be compensatory because it is not in keeping with the pH.

You then do a similar evaluation with the HCO_3^- (an alkalotic substance). If you have an acidosis with a low HCO_3^-, this must be a primary metabolic acidosis, of which the most common causes are renal and diabetic disease (both having a normal chloride and an elevated anion gap).

So the above example shows a metabolic acidosis with respiratory compensation (Kussmaul's breathing). Always consider the presence or absence of compensation. If absent, the changes are likely to be acute. You NEVER overcompensate.

Note that the elevated oxygen levels are a result of a lack of underlying respiratory disease and the patient being on oxygen therapy.

11a. T
11b. T
11c. F
11d. T
This is a metabolic alkalosis, the most common cause of which is prolonged vomiting, e.g. in bulimia. This will raise the pH, lower the K^+ and lower the chloride.

Other causes of a metabolic alkalosis include diuretic therapy and ingestion (accidental or otherwise) of an alkaline (e.g. bleach).

12a. F
12b. T
12c. T
12d. T
This is a primary respiratory alkalosis probably caused by high anxiety and resulting in hyperventilation. There is no evidence of metabolic (renal) HCO_3^- excretion in compensation as the bicarbonate is normal. The patient is likely to be experiencing tingling in the hands and feet as a result of the hyperventilation.

13a. F
13b. F
13c. F
13d. T
Alcohol ingestion, over a period of time, may result in haematological changes such as a raised MCV (mean corpuscular volume) and reduced platelets. However, acute changes include a raised serum uric acid level due to decreased urinary excretion of urate. The lactate:pyruvate ratio increases, which may result in mild acidosis on blood gas measurements. Hypoglycaemia often occurs following intoxication.

14a. T
14b. T
14c. T
14d. F
Lactic acid is produced by anaerobic metabolism in muscle and is oxidised to pyruvate (under aerobic conditions), which enters the tricarboxylic acid cycle as an energy substrate or is converted to glucose in the Cori (glucose–lactate) cycle in the liver (gluconeogenesis). High lactate essentially demonstrates underperfusion of tissues and will have a prognostic implication for settings such as trauma or sepsis. High levels of muscle activity, e.g. after a prolonged workout or a seizure, will result in elevated lactate levels. In the setting of sepsis, SIRS (systemic inflammatory response syndrome) plus prolonged hypotension (initial lactate >4.0 mmol/L or a repeat lactate after a fluid bolus of >2.0 mmol/L) is septic shock.

15a. F
15b. F
15c. F
15d. T
TSH is produced by the anterior pituitary under stimulation from hypothalamic TRH. T_4 (thyroxine) is the predominant thyroid hormone but T_3 (triiodothyronine) is more active. Most of the T_3 and T_4 is bound to TBG. Peripheral conversion of T_3 to T_4 occurs all over the body.

16a. T
16b. F
16c. T
16d. F
Parathyroid hormone is a peptide that results in increased osteoclastic activity in bone. This causes bone resorption, increasing the calcium level and lowering the phosphate levels. Parathyroid adenomas are associated with multiple endocrine neoplastic syndromes.

Renal vitamin D production is enhanced by parathyroid hormone.

17a. F
17b. F
17c. T
17d. T
Cortisol (similar to other glucocorticoid agents) has widespread actions that help restore homoeostasis after stress. It is secreted from the zona fasciculata with a diurnal biorhythm, with secretion being highest in the morning. Cortisol has the following major functions:

- It counteracts insulin by increasing gluconeogenesis, promoting breakdown of lipids (lipolysis) and proteins, and mobilising extrahepatic amino acids and ketone bodies.
- Cortisol raises the free amino acids in the serum. It does this by inhibiting collagen formation, decreasing amino acid uptake by muscle and inhibiting protein synthesis.

- It stimulates gastric acid secretion as well as acting as a diuretic hormone.
- Many copper enzymes are stimulated by cortisol, thereby increasing copper availability for immune purposes.
- Cortisol can weaken the activity of the immune system. It prevents proliferation of T cells by rendering the IL-2 producer T cells unresponsive to IL-1, and unable to produce the T-cell growth factor.
- Cortisol lowers bone formation, thus favouring the development of osteoporosis in the long term.
- It cooperates with adrenaline (epinephrine) to create memories of short-term emotional events; this is the proposed mechanism for storage of flashbulb memories.
- It increases blood pressure by increasing the sensitivity of the vasculature to adrenaline (epinephrine) and noradrenaline (norepinephrine). In the absence of cortisol, widespread vasodilatation occurs.
- It inhibits the secretion of corticotrophin-releasing hormone (CRH), resulting in feedback inhibition of ACTH (adrenocorticotrophic hormone or corticotrophin) secretion. Some researchers believe that this normal feedback system may become dysregulated when animals are exposed to chronic stress.
- It increases the effectiveness of catecholamines.
- It has anti-inflammatory effects mediated by reducing histamine secretion and stabilising lysosomal membranes.

18a. F
18b. T
18c. T
18d. F
Cushing's disease is usually caused by an ACTH-secreting pituitary tumour, resulting in cushingoid features and a high level of cortisol. Urinary cortisol is usually measured over a 24-hour period and the best screening test is the overnight dexamethasone suppression test.

19a. T
19b. T
19c. T
19d. F
Addison's disease is adrenocortical insufficiency. It may be autoimmune in nature and thus associated with other autoimmune diseases, e.g. type I diabetes and Graves' disease, but it may be the result of infection, e.g. TB, metastatic tumours or AIDS. There is underproduction of cortisol and aldosterone, resulting in a low glucose, low sodium and high potassium. Resultant ACTH levels are high to try to stimulate the gland. It is usually diagnosed by a short Synacthen test.

20a. F
20b. F
20c. T
20d. T
Conn's syndrome is hyperaldosteronism usually caused by an adrenal adenoma. There is usually high sodium and low potassium levels often

associated with hypertension, but the potassium may be normal in up to 30% of cases. Renin levels will be high to try to stimulate production of aldosterone.

21a. F
21b. T
21c. T
21d. F

Growth hormone (GH) is a polypeptide secreted in a pulsatile manner from the anterior pituitary. In addition to increasing height in children and adolescents, growth hormone has many other effects on the body:

- Increases calcium retention, and strengthens and increases the mineralisation of bone
- Increases muscle mass through sarcomere hyperplasia
- Promotes lipolysis
- Increases protein synthesis
- Stimulates the growth of all internal organs excluding the brain
- Plays a role in fuel homoeostasis
- Reduces liver uptake of glucose
- Promotes gluconeogenesis in the liver
- Contributes to the maintenance and function of pancreatic islets
- Stimulates the immune system.

Stimulators of GH secretion include:

- Growth hormone-releasing hormone (GHRH) from the arcuate nucleus in the hypothalamus
- Ghrelin, which is a hormone produced by cells lining the fundus of the stomach and ε cells of the pancreas; it stimulates appetite. Ghrelin levels rise before meals and fall after meals. It is the counter-regulatory hormone of leptin, which is produced by adipose tissue and induces satiation when present at higher levels
- Sleep
- Exercise
- Hypoglycaemia
- Dietary protein
- Increased androgen secretion during puberty
- Arginine (amino acid).

Inhibitors of GH secretion include:

- Somatostatin from the periventricular nucleus of the hypothalamus
- Circulating concentrations of GH and insulin-like growth factor 1 or IGF-1 (negative feedback on the pituitary and hypothalamus)
- Hyperglycaemia
- Glucocorticoids
- Estradiol or any oestrogen.

22a. T
22b. T
22c. F
22d. T
Renin is produced from the kidney in response to underperfusion of the juxtaglomerular cells and acts to convert angiotensinogen, which is produced in the liver, to angiotensin I.

Angiotensin-converting enzyme (ACE), in the lung, then converts this to the much more biologically active angiotensin II. Angiotensin II promotes salt and water retention in the kidney, raising blood pressure. It is also a potent vasoconstrictor and will stimulate the release of vasopressin and aldosterone.

23a. T
23b. T
23c. F
23d. T
Vitamin B_1 (thiamine) deficiency is associated with beriberi. This can be dry (polyneuropathy and loss of weight) or wet (cardiac failure). It usually occurs in people with chronic alcohol problems and is also associated with Wernicke–Korsakoff syndrome. Angular stomatitis is usually the result of iron deficiency.

24a. T
24b. F
24c. T
24d. F
Acute alcohol intoxication often results in hypoglycaemia. Acromegaly produces growth hormone, which antagonises insulin, resulting in hyperglycaemia. Acute pancreatitis often results in hyperglycaemia. Hepatocellular failure may cause hypoglycaemia as a result of reduced insulin levels.

25a. T
25b. F
25c. F
25d. T
The key here is the massively raised ALT, indicating an acute hepatitis.

1. Iron
   a. Most iron is absorbed in the ferrous (Fe^{2+}) state
   b. Iron absorption in the distal small bowel is reduced by proton pump inhibitors
   c. Iron absorption in the small bowel may be reduced by the ingestion of wheat
   d. Lead toxicity in children may lead to iron deficiency

2. Vitamin B_{12} deficiency
   a. Pernicious anaemia is the most common cause in the Western world
   b. Diseases of the terminal ileum may lead to vitamin B_{12} deficiency
   c. The Schilling test measures how much radioactive vitamin B_{12} has been absorbed into the bloodstream
   d. Anaemia caused by vitamin B_{12} deficiency may develop within months of gastric surgery

3. Folic acid
   a. Folic acid cannot be synthesised by humans
   b. Folic acid deficiency can cause placental abruption in pregnant women
   c. Deficiency is common in patients on long-term haemodialysis
   d. Folic acid deficiency is associated with malignancy

4. Sickle cell disease (SCD)
   a. There is a mutation on the α-haemoglobin chain
   b. The disease usually presents shortly after birth
   c. In an acute attack (crisis), a haemoglobin level of 9 g/dL would be a good prognostic indicator
   d. A megaloblastic anaemia is usually seen on blood analysis

5. Thalassaemia
   a. Elevated levels of HbF are common in β-thalassaemia
   b. α-Thalassaemia is most common in southern Europe
   c. Death is usually from features of severe anaemia
   d. A bone marrow transplantation may be curative

6. Pernicious anaemia
   a. Patients may present with absent ankle jerks
   b. It may be associated with Addison's disease
   c. It is treated with oral replacement of hydroxycobalamin (vitamin B_{12})
   d. Anaemia results from impaired synthesis of adenosine in marrow DNA

7. **Aplastic anaemia**
   a. Presentation may be with a thrombotic stroke
   b. Those patients with Fanconi's anaemia have an autoimmune aetiology
   c. Death may be secondary to sepsis
   d. Bone marrow transplantation is indicated in older patients

8. **Myeloproliferative disorders**
   a. They may present with fever, weight loss and splenomegaly
   b. Essential thrombocythaemia often presents with bleeding
   c. Chronic lymphocytic leukaemia is one type of myeloproliferative disorder
   d. Myelofibrosis is associated with teardrop cells on blood film analysis

9. **Regarding the ESR test**
   a. This is a test that measures the rate of sedimentation of red cells over 1 minute
   b. In patients with malignancy, the red cells stick to each other and sediment much more slowly
   c. The ESR generally rises with age and is usually higher in men
   d. The ESR is usually low in patients with polycythaemia

10. **Factor V Leiden mutation thrombophilia**
    a. This is an autosomal recessive disorder leading to a hypercoagulable state
    b. Those heterozygous for the abnormal gene are usually unaffected
    c. Presentation is usually with bleeding gums
    d. Females with the condition have an increased risk of myocardial infarction if taking combined oral contraceptives

11. **Haemophilia A**
    a. This is an inherited condition usually seen in young girls
    b. The bleeding time is usually normal
    c. Patients with this condition will usually have excessive bleeding after tooth extraction
    d. NSAID therapy should be avoided

12. **The clotting cascade**
    a. Vitamin K is required for the hepatic synthesis of factor X
    b. Both the intrinsic and extrinsic pathways result in the activation of factor IX
    c. Heparin prevents the formation of thrombin
    d. Warfarin reduces the synthesis of factor V

13. **Acute lymphoblastic leukaemia**
    a. It is the most common paediatric malignancy
    b. It is more common in girls
    c. It peaks at the age range 2–5 years in children
    d. The malignant cells are usually Sudan black positive

14. **Acute myeloid leukaemia (AML)**
    a. The presence of Auer rods on blood film is pathognomonic
    b. Myeloblasts in the blood film are usually PAS positive
    c. Lymphadenopathy is common
    d. Patients may present with gum hypertrophy

15. **Chronic lymphocytic leukaemia (CLL)**
    a. Most patients are young
    b. Lymphadenopathy is common
    c. Treatment with chemotherapy usually starts shortly after diagnosis
    d. Most cases involve T cells

16. **Multiple myeloma**
    a. A bone marrow aspirate shows excess plasma cells
    b. Monoclonal bands are usually IgM
    c. Bence Jones proteins are found on serum electrophoresis
    d. A common presentation is often renal failure

17. **Prothrombin time**
    a. The correct blood tube to measure this is one containing EDTA
    b. The prothrombin time is a measure of the extrinsic clotting pathway
    c. It is often referred to as the INR
    d. It is raised in von Willebrand's disease

18. **Regarding the partial thromboplastin time**
    a. A normal range is 10–15 seconds
    b. It is a measure of the intrinsic clotting pathway
    c. It is raised in patients receiving warfarin
    d. It is raised in haemophilia A

19. **Disseminated intravascular coagulation**
    a. This may be triggered by malignancy
    b. The INR is elevated
    c. Schistocytes are seen on a blood film
    d. The platelet count will be elevated

20. **Warfarin**
    a. This produces vitamin K deficiency
    b. It has a half-life of approximately 5 hours
    c. It may result in an elevated aPTT
    d. It is teratogenic

21. **Hodgkin's lymphoma**
    a. The characteristic cell seen on biopsy is the Reed–Sternberg cell
    b. Patients with this condition often have painful lymphadenopathy
    c. The presence of systemic symptoms improves the prognosis
    d. Women are more likely to have the disease than men

22. **Non-Hodgkin's lymphoma**
    a. The incidence has increased over the last 20 years
    b. It is usually a T-cell malignancy
    c. Patients tend to present late with extranodal disease
    d. Burkitt's lymphoma is more common in HIV-positive individuals

23. **Hyperviscosity syndrome**
    a. The microcirculation is impaired
    b. It may present with genitourinary bleeding
    c. It may present with visual loss
    d. Plasmapheresis may be a suitable treatment

24. **Protein S deficiency**
    a. Protein S is a vitamin K-dependent anticoagulant protein
    b. It is associated with fetal loss in women
    c. It may be an acquired disorder
    d. It usually results in GI bleeding

25. **Antiphospholipid syndrome**
    a. It is more common in women
    b. Most patients will also have SLE
    c. There is an increased risk of acute myocardial infarction
    d. Adrenal insufficiency may be the presenting feature

7. Haematology: Answers

1a. F
1b. F
1c. T
1d. T

Iron can be ingested organically as haem iron, found in meat, or as inorganic iron in either the ferrous (Fe^{2+}) or the ferric (Fe^{3+}) state. Iron is absorbed in the duodenum in the oxidised Fe^{3+} state and this is affected by gastric pH. Antacids will prevent oxidisation and hence reduce iron absorption. Once absorbed, it binds to transferrin, which delivers it to its cellular targets. Ascorbate and citrate increase iron uptake, by acting as weak chelators to help to solubilise the metal in the duodenum. Conversely, iron absorption is inhibited by plant phytates and tannins. These compounds also chelate iron, but prevent its uptake by the absorption machinery. Phytates are prominent in wheat and some other cereals, whereas tannins are prevalent in (non-herbal) teas. Lead blocks iron metabolism through competitive inhibition. Further, lead interferes with a number of important iron-dependent metabolic steps such as haem biosynthesis. This has severe consequences in children, and iron deficiency may develop in areas where the lead content of the soil and water is high.

2a. T
2b. T
2c. F
2d. F

Vitamin B_{12} deficiency leads to a macrocytic (raised MCV – mean corpuscular volume) anaemia. Causes of macrocytosis without anaemia include drugs (alcohol, zidovudine/AZT), liver disease, pregnancy and hypothyroidism. The most common cause of vitamin B_{12} deficiency in the West is pernicious anaemia (lack of intrinsic factor). Vitamin B_{12} is found in all animal cells, especially the liver, and absorption occurs in the terminal ileum after it has bound to intrinsic factor, which is produced in the gastric parietal cells. The human body stores enough vitamin B_{12} for at least 3–4 years. Schilling's test is used to differentiate the cause of vitamin B_{12} deficiency. A small radioactive dose of oral vitamin B_{12} is given and the urine is measured for radioactivity. The process is then repeated after an oral dose of intrinsic factor. This should therefore show whether the deficiency is due to lack of intrinsic factor (pernicious anaemia) or malabsorption in the terminal ileum. It is necessary to saturate the body stores first with an intramuscular dose of vitamin B_{12}.

3a. T
3b. T
3c. T
3d. T

Folic acid is composed of a pterin ring connected to p-aminobenzoic acid (PABA) and conjugated with one or more glutamate residues. PABA cannot be synthesised by humans; hence our folic acid must be obtained from our diet.

Folate is distributed widely in green leafy vegetables, citrus fruits and animal products. Causes of a low folate include poor diet (people with alcohol problems), pregnancy, haemolysis, malignancy, malabsorption (coeliac disease, tropical sprue), drugs (phenytoin, trimethoprim) and haemodialysis. Possible pregnancy complications secondary to maternal folate status may include spontaneous abortion, abruptio placentae and congenital malformations (e.g. neural tube defect). Although the exact mechanism is not understood, a relative folate shortage may exacerbate an underlying genetic predisposition to neural tube defects. Folic acid deficiency is associated with an increased risk of colon cancer.

4a. F
4b. F
4c. T
4d. T
HbS arises from a mutation substituting thymine for adenine in the sixth codon of the β-chain gene (GAG to GTG). These changes are responsible for the profound clinical expressions of the sickling syndromes that occur when the oxygen tension falls.

SCD usually manifests early in childhood. For the first 6 months of life, infants are protected by high levels of HbF.

Three poor prognostic factors are:

1. Dactylitis in infants younger than 1 year
2. Hb level <7 g/dL
3. Leukocytosis in the absence of infection.

Chronic haemolysis leads to folate deficiency and a megaloblastic picture on the blood film.

5a. T
5b. F
5c. F
5d. T
The thalassaemias are inherited disorders of haemoglobin (Hb) synthesis. Their clinical severity varies widely, ranging from asymptomatic forms to severe and fatal syndromes. A decrease in the rate of production of a certain globin chain or chains (α, β, γ, δ) impedes Hb synthesis and creates an imbalance with the other, normally produced globin chains. The abnormal Hb precipitates, resulting in severe anaemia.

Hb	Peptide chains	Percentage adult blood	Percentage fetal blood
HbA	$\alpha_2\beta_2$	97	10–50
HbA$_2$	$\alpha_2\delta_2$	2.5	Trace
HbF	$\alpha_2\gamma_2$	0.5	50–90

Hence in β-thalassaemia HbA_2 and HbF are elevated because HbA will be faulty and precipitate. β-Thalassaemia is common in southern Europe, the Middle East, India and Africa. α-Thalassaemia is more common in South-East Asia. Patients require life-long transfusions and death is usually from features of iron overload. Megaloblastic anaemia often develops as a result of folate deficiency. Bone marrow transplantations may be curative in selected patients.

6a. T
6b. T
6c. F
6d. F
Pernicious anaemia (PA) results from a lack of intrinsic factor leading to malabsorption of vitamin B_{12}. It affects the central nervous system (CNS), peripheral nerves, gut and the tongue. Common features include weakness, tiredness, shortness of breath (SOB), paraesthesias, glossitis, diarrhoea and weight loss. Signs include splenomegaly, retinal haemorrhages and fever. It is often associated with vitiligo, Addison's disease, thyroid disease and carcinoma of the stomach. Anaemia develops as a result of defective methionine synthesis.

Neurological features may occur in the absence of anaemia and include:

- Subacute combined degeneration of the spinal cord
- Peripheral neuropathy
- Loss of vibration/joint position sense (dorsal columns)
- Extensor plantar responses
- Brisk knee jerks
- Absent ankle jerks.

The MCV is elevated and white cells and platelets often reduced. Treatment is intramuscular replacement of hydroxycobalamin. Neurological signs often recover.

7a. F
7b. F
7c. T
7d. F
Aplastic anaemia results from marrow failure. All three cell lines are affected so patients are anaemic, thrombocytopenic and neutropenic. It is frequently secondary to viral infections (often transient) but may be drug induced, inherited (Fanconi's anaemia) or autoimmune. Cytotoxic drugs are an iatrogenic cause. Treatment is usually supportive but, in the young healthy population, bone marrow transplantation may be a treatment option.

8a. T
8b. T
8c. F
8d. T
Myeloproliferative disorders are the result of the uncontrolled differentiation of the myeloid precursors. These include erythrocytes (polycythaemia rubra

vera), white blood cells (chronic myeloid leukaemia), platelets (thrombo-cythaemia) and fibroblasts (myelofibrosis).

They have common features such as fever, weight loss, malaise, itching and splenomegaly. In essential thrombocythaemia, although the cell numbers are large, they are dysmorphic and dysfunctional, leading to bleeding as a common presentation.

9a. F
9b. F
9c. F
9d. T
The ESR (erythrocyte sedimentation rate) is a measure of the sedimentation of red cells in anticoagulated blood over 1 hour.

In the presence of certain diseases (inflammatory, malignancy, connective tissue, infection) the red cells become coated with surface proteins, causing them to stick together and they fall (sediment) much quicker; hence the ESR is raised. In general, the ESR increases with age and anaemia. As a general rule the normal ESR is age/2 for men and (age+10)/2 for women.

The ESR is low in polycythaemia, in sickle cell disease and in those with cryoglobulinaemia.

10a. F
10b. F
10c. F
10d. T
Factor V Leiden mutation is a rare autosomal dominant condition resulting in thrombophilia. Most patients are heterozygous for the condition and present with venous thromboembolism. The risk is increased even further for those on oestrogen-containing contraceptives and HRT, but the risk still remains low and general screening is not indicated.

11a. F
11b. T
11c. T
11d. T
Haemophilia A (factor VIII deficiency) is an X-linked disorder usually affecting males, the females being carriers for the condition. Some females may be affected depending on the degree of lyonisation (a process by which one of the two copies of the X chromosome present in females is inactivated). Usually, the activated partial thromboplastin time (aPTT) is prolonged; however, a normal aPTT does not exclude mild or even moderate haemophilia. Severe haemophilia is easily identified with a significantly prolonged aPTT. Bleeding times, prothrombin times and platelet counts are normal. Patients often present with bleeding (skin, gums, joints). Treatment is usually with either desmopressin (which increases factor VIII level) or factor VIII replacement, depending on the severity of the bleed.

Intramuscular injections and NSAIDs should be avoided in these patients, as should aspiration of haemarthroses.

12a. T
12b. F
12c. T
12d. F
The clotting cascade has an intrinsic (factors XII, XI and IX) and an extrinsic pathway (tissue factor) that both result in activation of the Stuart–Prower factor X. This, in turn, together with calcium, phospholipid and factor V, converts prothrombin to thrombin, which then results in the conversion of fibrinogen to fibrin. Heparin is an antithrombin agent.

Warfarin inhibits the synthesis of factors II, VII, IX and X.

13a. T
13b. F
13c. T
13d. F
In ALL (acute lymphoblastic leukaemia) there is malignant transformation of the lymphoblast, which infiltrates the marrow (resulting in failure), and the lymphoblasts are often seen on the peripheral blood film.

It is the most common malignancy seen in children and is more common in boys. It peaks in incidence at 2–5 years. It often presents with anaemia, thrombocytopenia and leukopenia.

Bone pain is common and in T-cell disease there is often a mediastinal mass seen on the chest radiograph. The lymphoblasts stain negative for Sudan black and peroxidase, but stain positive with PAS (periodic acid–Schiff). Initial treatment to induce remission is chemotherapy with prednisolone and vincristine. Intrathecal methotrexate is also commonly used. Cure rates of up to 80% have been described.

Poor prognostic factors include:

- Counts >20 000 at presentation
- Age <2 or >10 years
- Males
- Those with an associated chromosomal defect
- T-cell disease.

14a. T
14b. F
14c. F
14d. T
In AML there is malignant proliferation of the myeloblast in the blood and marrow. Presentation is usually with symptoms and signs of bone marrow failure and/or DIC (disseminated intravascular coagulation).

Hepatosplenomegaly is common, whereas lymphadenopathy is rare. Gum infiltration is common. The myeloblasts stain positive with Sudan black and peroxidase, but negative for PAS. Auer rods when seen are pathognomonic for AML. Treatment is with chemotherapy and bone marrow transplantation in young children. Neuronal disease is unusual and intrathecal methotrexate is rarely required. Prognosis is generally poor.

15a. F
15b. T
15c. F
15d. F
CLL is a low-grade malignancy of small lymphocytes that is common in elderly people. There is usually a gradual onset of fatigue, malaise and lymphadeno-pathy. B-cell disease is by far the most common and hypogammaglobulinaemia occurs in up to a third of patients. CLL is incurable and chemotherapy may be started for late symptomatic disease.

16a. T
16b. F
16c. F
16d. T
Multiple myeloma is a B-cell malignancy of the plasma cells. These proliferate in the marrow, resulting in failure. There is usually a decreased albumin level and increased protein levels as a result of high immunoglobulins, which on electrophoresis are usually IgG. IgM is the rarest form. Light chains are precipitated in the urine (Bence Jones proteins). Bone destruction with lytic lesions is common and results in hypercalcaemia, which may lead to renal failure (also caused by hyperuricaemia, urinary tract infections and light chain precipitation). Neurological problems often occur secondary to plasmacyto-mas. The ESR is usually extremely high. Treatment is usually symptomatic with radiotherapy for bone pain.

17a. F
17b. T
17c. T
17d. F
The INR (international normalised ratio or prothrombin time) is a measure of the extrinsic pathway of the clotting cascade and is measured in a bottle containing sodium citrate.

It is elevated in vitamin K deficiency, liver disease, DIC and coumarin therapy, i.e. warfarin.

18a. F
18b. T
18c. F
18d. T
The partial thromboplastin time (PTT) is sometimes referred to as the kaolin cephalin clotting time (KCCT) or aPTT, and is usually 35–45 seconds. It is a measure of the intrinsic clotting cascade and is increased in heparin therapy, DIC and haemophilia.

19a. T
19b. T
19c. T
19d. F
DIC is the pathological activation of coagulation leading to haemolysis, with consumption of platelets and clotting factors.

Common triggers are malignancy, infection and trauma. The patient usually presents with extensive bruising and bleeding, and organ failure usually ensues. The INR and aPTT are raised, and platelets and fibrinogen are decreased (consumption). A blood film will demonstrate fragmented red cells (schistocytes). Treatment involves platelets and fresh frozen plasma.

20a. F
20b. F
20c. T
20d. T
Warfarin is a coumarin derivative that works by preventing vitamin K epoxide reductase, thus rendering vitamin K inactive. It does not produce vitamin K deficiency. It affects clotting factors II, VII, IX and X, and so greatly affects the INR but it also has some effect on the extrinsic pathway via inhibition of factor IX; hence the aPTT may be raised. It has an elimination half-life of 40–70 hours, and that is why, if immediate anticoagulation is required, heparin should be used. It should be avoided in the first trimester of pregnancy because it is teratogenic.

21a. T
21b. F
21c. F
21d. F
Hodgkin's lymphoma is a malignancy of Reed–Sternberg lymphocytes. It affects young adults and elderly people and is more common in men. It usually presents with painless lymphadenopathy, the neck being the most common site. It may present with constitutional symptoms such as weight loss, night sweats and fever, which would worsen the prognosis for any classification group, as would a raised ESR and the presence of anaemia.

Hypercalcaemia is common and in late disease hepatosplenomegaly may be present.

Diagnosis is usually based on lymph node biopsy, and Ann Arbor staging depends on where the disease is identified:

Stage I: confined to a single region
Stage II: confined to two regions on the same side as the diaphragm
Stage III: disease both sides of the diaphragm
Stage IV: extra-lymph node disease.

The cell type is also of prognostic significance. Nodular sclerosing, mixed cellularity and lymphocyte predominant have relatively good prognoses but lymphocyte-depleted disease has a poor prognosis.

22a. T
22b. F
22c. T
22d. T
Non-Hodgkin's disease includes all lymphomas that do not have the Reed–Sternberg cell. There are usually B-cell types and generally they have a much poorer prognosis, because they tend to present late with extranodal disease. The incidence is increasing possibly as a result of increased exposure to HIV, EBV (Epstein–Barr virus) and sunlight.

23a. T
23b. T
23c. T
23d. T
As the plasma viscosity rises, the microcirculation is impaired as a result of sludging. Hyperviscosity is seen in malignancy, especially myeloma, Waldenström's macroglobulinaemia and polycythaemia rubra vera. It usually presents as visual disturbances (retinal haemorrhages), headaches and either gastrointestinal or genitourinary bleeding. Treatment involves either phlebotomy or plasmapheresis.

24a. T
24b. T
24c. T
24d. F
Protein S is a vitamin K-dependent anticoagulant protein. Its major function is as a cofactor to facilitate the action of activated protein C. Protein S deficiencies are associated with thrombosis. Protein S deficiency may be hereditary (autosomal dominant inheritance) or acquired (hepatic disease or a vitamin K deficiency). It usually manifests clinically as venous thromboembolism but is also associated with fetal loss in women. There is little or no association with arterial thromboembolism.

25a. T
25b. F
25c. T
25d. T
Antiphospholipid syndrome is a disorder characterised by recurrent venous or arterial thrombosis and/or fetal losses associated with characteristic laboratory abnormalities, such as persistently elevated levels of antibodies directed against membrane anionic phospholipids (e.g. anticardiolipin antibody or lupus anticoagulant). It can be associated with other rheumatological disorders, e.g. SLE (systemic lupus erythematosus) but this is not common. It is more common in women.

The adrenal gland is prone to infarction (and even haemorrhage) and may be the presenting feature.

8. Pathology: Questions

1. C-reactive protein
a. This is made in the bone marrow of long bones
b. It is produced in response to increased levels of interleukin 6
c. It activates the complement system
d. Levels will be elevated in viral infections

2. In anaphylactoid reactions
a. Mast cells degranulate, releasing histamine
b. The allergen binds to IgE
c. Diarrhoea may be a presenting feature
d. Steroids may prevent further relapse

3. Concerning meningitis
a. Meningococcal meningitis is the most common type in adults in the UK
b. Treatment with steroids may benefit those with severe meningococcal disease
c. There has been a decline in the incidence of *Haemophilus influenzae* meningitis in pre-school children
d. Meningitic symptoms in a patient with meningococcal sepsis will improve the prognosis

4. Regarding immunoglubulins
a. IgE is secreted by mast cells
b. IgA is present in breast milk
c. IgG is usually the first immunoglobulin produced after an infection
d. IgG may cross the placenta

5. HIV may be transmitted by the following routes
a. Mosquito bite
b. Ingestion of urine
c. Breastfeeding
d. Human bites

6. In myocarditis
a. The ESR is usually raised
b. The most common ECG abnormality is ST depression
c. It may be caused by HIV
d. It may present with sudden death

7. **In the treatment of needle-stick injuries**
   a. HIV post-exposure prophylaxis (PEP) is recommended to be given within 24 hours
   b. Where the donor has unknown HIV status, PEP is not recommended
   c. Interferon as PEP is recommended when the donor status is known to be positive for hepatitis C
   d. A recent titre of >100 mIU/mL of antibody to the hepatitis B surface antigen (HBsAg) in the recipient suggests hepatitis B immunity and does not require anti-HB immunoglobulin in a HBsAg-positive needle-stick injury donor

8. **In viral hepatitis**
   a. One may be immunised against hepatitis A
   b. Hepatitis E is transmitted primarily via the faecal–oral route
   c. Up to 50% of those with hepatitis C progress to cirrhosis
   d. Hepatitis A may be contracted by swimming in infected water

9. **Rheumatoid factor**
   a. This is an autoantibody directed towards IgG
   b. It is associated with Sjögren's syndrome
   c. It is a good marker for disease progression in arthritis
   d. It may be present in cases of SLE

10. **The following antibodies are correctly matched to their associated disease**
    a. Anti-nuclear antibodies and SLE
    b. Rheumatoid factor and leprosy
    c. Anti-mitochondrial antibodies and Wegner's granulomatosis
    d. Anti-neutrophil cytoplasmic antibodies and primary biliary cirrhosis

11. **The following are recognised pulmonary complication of AIDS**
    a. Aspergilloma
    b. Kaposi's sarcoma
    c. Bacterial lobar pneumonia
    d. Fibrosing alveolitis

12. **Concerning urinary tract infections**
    a. They are more common in men
    b. In young men they usually represent a sexually transmitted infection
    c. They should always be investigated by imaging of the renal tract in pre-school children
    d. The most common causative organism is *E. coli*

13. **Concerning malaria**
    a. Mosquito nets help to reduce infection rates
    b. Quinine is mainly used for malaria prophylaxis
    c. Cerebral malaria responds well to steroids
    d. The diagnosis is usually made on clinical grounds

14. **When a wound heals by primary intention**
    a. The wound space fills with clot and exudates in the first 24 hours
    b. Epithelial cells migrate over the surface skin and proliferate in the wound
    c. Capillary sprouts are seen by the end of day 1
    d. Vascularity of a scar will decrease with time

15. **Pelvic inflammatory disease**
    a. The most common causative organism is *N. gonorrhoeae*
    b. It may be contracted after termination of a pregnancy
    c. It results in a higher incidence of ectopic pregnancy
    d. It may result in peritonitis

16. **Gas gangrene**
    a. It is usually caused by infection with *Clostridium perfringens*
    b. The incubation period is often longer than a week
    c. Treatment may include hyperbaric oxygen
    d. The absence of radiological soft tissue gas excludes the diagnosis

8. Pathology: Answers

1a. F
1b. T
1c. T
1d. T

C-reactive protein (CRP) is produced in the liver and binds to phosphocholine receptors on microbes; this activates the complement system. It is an acute phase inflammatory marker that is produced as a result of increased levels of IL-6. It may be used to monitor disease progression, and will be elevated in viral infections, but tends to be higher with bacterial infections.

2a. T
2b. F
2c. T
2d. T

In anaphylactic reactions the antigen binds to IgE, resulting in mast cell and basophil degranulation, which releases histamine and other chemotactic substances including prostaglandins, leukotrienes and cytokines. The complement system is activated. An anaphylactoid reaction results in exactly the same clinical scenario but is not mediated by IgE. Typically these result in cardiovascular collapse, rash and airway compromise, but it may affect any system via H_1- and H_2-receptors, e.g. in the gut, resulting in diarrhoea. There is typically a biphasic response.

Intramuscular adrenaline (epinephrine) 0.5 mL of 1/1000 is the treatment for airway compromise or hypotension together with intravenous fluids and antihistamines. Always remove the offending antigen if possible, e.g. bee sting. The second or late phase is responsive to treatment with steroids.

3a. F
3b. F
3c. T
3d. T

Causes of meningitis are age dependent. In order of frequency they are:

First month: *Escherichia coli*, group B streptococci and *Listeria* spp.
Second month: group B streptococci.
Older than 2 months: *Streptococcus pneumoniae* and *Neisseria meningitidis* currently cause most of the cases of bacterial meningitis; *Haemophilus influenzae* may still occur, especially in children who have not received the Hib vaccine.
Adults: *S. pneumoniae*, *H. influenzae*, *N. meningitidis*, Gram-negative bacilli, staphylococci, streptococci and *Listeria* spp.

Steroids are said to improve the outcome in those patients with pneumococcal disease if given before antibiotics but they are not advised in meningococcal disease. Meningococcal septicaemia has a poor prognosis, which is worse in those without meningitic symptoms.

4a. F
4b. T
4c. F
4d. T
The following table summarises the actions of different immunoglobulins:

Name	Description
IgA	Found in mucosal areas, such as the gut, respiratory tract and genitourinary tract, preventing colonisation by pathogens
	It is also found in breast milk, saliva and tears
IgD	This is an antigen receptor on B cells that have not been exposed to antigens
IgE	Binds to allergens and triggers histamine release from mast cells and basophils
IgG	This provides most of the antibody-based immunity against invading pathogens
	It is the only antibody capable of crossing the placenta to give passive immunity to the fetus
IgM	Expressed on the surface of B cells and in a secreted form with very high avidity
	Eliminates pathogens in the early stages of B-cell-mediated (humoral) immunity before there is sufficient IgG

5a. F
5b. F
5c. T
5d. T
Human immunodeficiency virus (HIV) is usually transmitted by exchange of body fluids. Mosquito bites do not result in seroconversion, because the direction of blood is always away from the individual. There are case reports of transmission of HIV through human bites where the skin has been broken. Urine and tears are not considered infectious.

6a. T
6b. F
6c. T
6d. T
Myocarditis is acute inflammation of the myocardium. It may present with chest pain, arrhythmia, cardiac failure or sudden death. It has many causes including viral, bacterial, fungal and parasitic infections, as well as electric shocks and radiotherapy. Inflammatory markers are usually raised and the most common ECG abnormality is T-wave inversion.

7a. F
7b. T
7c. F
7d. T
PEP is recommended within 1 hour if the donor is known to be HIV positive. Interferon is not recommended as prophylaxis but is effective only in the treatment of an established case of hepatitis C. More than 10 mIU/mL of antibody to HBsAg indicates a response to vaccination and therefore immunoglobulin is not required.

8a. T
8b. T
8c. T
8d. T
Hepatitis A and E are transmitted via the faecal–oral route. It rarely results in serious liver problems and can be immunised against. Other viral causes of viral hepatitis are spread by intravenous crossover or sharing of body fluids. Only 10% of those with hepatitis B progress to cirrhosis although it may be up to 50% for hepatitis C.

9a. T
9b. T
9c. F
9d. T
Rheumatoid factor (RF) is an autoantibody directed towards the Fc portion of IgG. It is positively associated with both rheumatoid arthritis and Sjögren's syndrome and other autoimmune disorders. It is a poor marker for monitoring disease progression.

10a. T
10b. T
10c. F
10d. F

ANA (anti-nuclear antibody)	SLE
	Systemic sclerosis
	Sjögren's syndrome
	Chronic active hepatitis
	Primary biliary cirrhosis
RF (rheumatoid factor)	Rheumatoid arthritis
	Sjögren's syndrome
	SLE
	Systemic sclerosis
	Viral hepatitis
	Leprosy
	TB

(continued)

Anti-mitochondrial antibody	Chronic active hepatitis
	Primary biliary cirrhosis
	Cryptogenic cirrhosis
	Syphilis
Smooth muscle antibody	Chronic active hepatitis
	Primary biliary cirrhosis
	Sclerosing cholangitis
	Pulmonary hypertension
ANCA (anti-neutrophil cytoplasmic antibody)	Wegner's granulomatosis
	Churg–Strauss syndrome
	Polyarteritis nodosa

11a. T
11b. T
11c. T
11d. F
Patients with AIDS are prone to both common and unusual respiratory problems. Unusual infections include cytomegalovirus, cryptococci, tuberculosis, aspergilloma and *Pneumocystis* sp. Kaposi's sarcoma may affect the skin, lung tissue or bowel.

12a. F
12b. T
12c. T
12d. T
UTIs are more common in women due to a short urethra. People with diabetes and men with an enlarged prostate are also at risk. In children, one should always look for abnormalities of the renal tract. In young adults, the aetiology is usually that of a sexually transmitted infection, and these patients should be treated by the genitourinary medicine (GUM) department.

13a. T
13b. F
13c. F
13d. F
Mosquito nets do help to reduce the transmission of malaria by reducing the number of bites. Quinine is a drug used only for treatment of established disease but resistance is increasing. Other therapeutic drugs include primaquine. Prophylactic drugs include proguanil and chloroquine. Cerebral malaria may result in an increase in cerebral pressure but mortality is increased in those treated with steroids. The diagnosis is usually made by examination of blood films.

14a. T
14b. T
14c. F
14d. T
In the first 24 hours the wound fills with clot and exudates and is invaded by neutrophils and monocytes as a result of inflammatory changes. Epithelial cells migrate to and proliferate in the wound. By the end of the first day, mitoses in the connective tissue are seen and by day 3 capillary sprouts are seen. Reticulin fibres are present by day 4 or 5 and these are usually strong enough to take any strain by about 8–10 days, which is when most sutures are removed.

The initial scar is usually highly vascular (pink) but becomes less so with time (old scars appear white). A wound may take weeks to develop its full strength.

15a. F
15b. T
15c. T
15d. T
Ninety per cent of cases of pelvic inflammatory disease (PID) occur as a result of the sexual transmission of organisms that may infect the cervix, uterus, fallopian tubes and even the abdomen. The most common organism is *Chlamydia trachomatis*, although *N. gonorrhoeae* and *Mycoplasma* spp. are other causes. It may be contracted after termination of pregnancy or evacuation of retained products. Ectopic pregnancy is five times more common in this group and chlamydial infection may lead to infertility.

16a. T
16b. F
16c. T
16d. F
Gas gangrene is due to the rapidly progressive infection with *Clostridium perfringens* (Gram-positive bacillus). The incubation is typically 4 days but is often less and may be merely hours. It usually presents with pain in a wound or muscle but rapidly spreads to other tissues and may eventually lead to septic shock. Gas is often seen on radiographs but the absence of gas does not exclude the diagnosis. Treatment involves antibiotics, debridement and hyperbaric oxygen.

1. The following results were obtained from a randomised controlled trial of a new test, 'FRB', in the detection of heart failure

	Heart failure	
	Present	Absent
FRB-positive	80	20
FRB-negative	120	180

   a. The sensitivity of FRB in the diagnosis of heart failure is 40% (80/200)
   b. The specificity of FRB in the diagnosis of heart failure is 10% (20/200)
   c. The positive predictive value of FRB in the diagnosis of heart failure is 20% (20/100)
   d. The negative predictive value of FRB in the diagnosis of heart failure is 60% (180/300)

2. Regarding blinding in clinical trials
   a. In a 'double-blind' clinical trial, neither the investigator nor the patients are aware of which intervention they are being given
   b. Blinding helps to reduce publication bias
   c. Clinical trials that are not blinded are worthless
   d. In a double-blind trial those interpreting the data may know which treatment a patient was given without compromising the results

3. When describing the results of trials and reviews
   a. The number needed to treat (NNT) is the reciprocal of the odds ratio
   b. In therapy trials the higher the NNT the more effective the therapy
   c. In therapy trials the higher the number needed to harm the better the therapy
   d. A drug with a NNT of 10 is useless

4. The normal distribution
   a. This is used to describe parametric data
   b. Of the measurements, 99% lie within 2 standard deviations of the mean
   c. The mean describes the peak of the curve
   d. It can be symmetrical or asymmetrical

5. The following data were obtained from a trial comparing the drug Georgium with placebo in the treatment of acute pain, where success is defined as a 50% reduction in pain scores at 24 hours

	50% reduction in pain	
Drug given	Present	Absent
Georgium	70	30
Placebo	20	80

  a. The control event rate (CER) is 20/80
  b. The experimental event rate (EER) is 70/100
  c. The absolute risk reduction is: Experimental event rate (EER) – Control event rate (CER)
  d. Georgium is better than placebo at achieving a 50% reduction in pain

6. Which of the following are commonly used statistical tests?
  a. The χ^2 test
  b. Student's t-test
  c. The Mann–Whitney test
  d. Fisher's exact test

7. The following are the results of a trial using Jasarch, a newly discovered protein in blood, that may be useful in the diagnosis of sarcoid

	Sarcoid	
Jasarch	Present	Absent
Positive	70	130
Negative	30	120

  a. The sensitivity of Jasarch in the diagnosis of sarcoid = 70/200 = 35%
  b. The specificity of Jasarch in the diagnosis of sarcoid = 120/150 = 80%
  c. The positive predictive value of Jasarch in the diagnosis of sarcoid is 70/100 = 70%
  d. The negative predictive value of Jasarch in the diagnosis of sarcoid is 120/250 = 48%

8. **Likelihood ratios**
   a. A likelihood ratio describes the ratio of positive to negative tests
   b. A positive likelihood ratio of 1 indicates that the test is of no clinical utility
   c. Likelihood ratios can be used to convert a pre-test probability to a post-test probability
   d. Likelihood ratios are a clinical application of Bayes' theorem

9. **Regarding confidence intervals when analysing data from a clinical trial**
   a. A 95% confidence interval gives a range around the trial data within which we can be 95% sure that the true value lies
   b. The narrower the confidence interval the more likely that the trial result is true
   c. A 95% confidence interval is calculated as 2 standard deviations either side of the trial result
   d. Confidence intervals assume the use of parametric data

10. **Regarding potential errors in a study**
    a. The probability of a type 1 error is the same as the significance level
    b. If the sample size stays the same, reducing the chance of a type 1 error will increase the chance of a type 2 error
    c. Assuming that all other conditions stay the same, reducing the sample size will always increase the chance of both type 1 and type 2 errors
    d. Type 1 error (α) is the rejection of the null hypothesis when it is true

9. Statistics: Answers

1a. T
1b. F
1c. F
1d. T
The results of diagnosis trials are usually presented in the form of a 2×2 table and described using sensitivity, specificity, positive and negative predictive values:

	Target disorder	
	Present	**Absent**
FRB-positive	$a = 80$	$b = 20$
FRB-negative	$c = 120$	$d = 180$

Sensitivity $= a/(a+c) = 80/200 = 40\%$
Specificity $= d/(b+d) = 180/200 = 90\%$
Positive predictive value $= a/(a+b) = 80/100 = 80\%$
Negative predictive value $= d/(c+d) = 180/300 = 60\%$.

2a. T
2b. F
2c. F
2d. F
In a 'double-blind' trial, neither the investigators nor the patients are aware of the treatment given. It is also important that those analysing the data are unaware of the intervention given to each participant. Although blinding is desirable in clinical trials, with the aim of making the results more objective, it is sometimes not possible (especially in emergency medicine). For example, it would be impossible to blind patients and investigators when comparing non-invasive ventilation and medical therapy. Publication bias is the publication of trials, by researchers, pharmaceutical companies and journals, that are positive rather than negative.

3a. F
3b. F
3c. T
3d. F
The number needed to treat (NNT) is the inverse of the absolute risk reduction (ARR), or 1/ARR, and is a useful way to describe the effectiveness of a treatment. The lower the NNT the better; a therapy with an NNT of 1 would be ideal but rarely occurs. A NNT of 5–20 is much more usual and still represents a good therapeutic benefit (thrombolysis in acute myocardial infarction has an NNT of somewhere between 8 and 20). The number needed to harm (NNH) is similar but represents the adverse effects from a therapy. Here the higher the number the better.

4a. T
4b. F
4c. T
4d. F
The normal, or Gaussian, distributions are a family of distributions that have the same basic symmetrical shape. The nature of the shape is determined by the mean, at the peak of the curve, and the standard deviation, which describes the shape or girth of the curve. Within a normal distribution 95% of the observations lie within 2 standard deviations of the mean; 99.7% lie within 3 standard deviations.

5a. F
5b. T
5c. T
5d. T

Drug given	50% reduction in pain	
	Present	**Absent**
Georgium	70	30
Placebo	20	80

Here the control event rate (CER) = 20/100 = 0.2 (20%)
The experimental event rate (EER) = 70/100 = 0.7 (70%)
The absolute risk reduction (ARR) = EER − CER = 0.7 − 0.2 = 0.5 (50%)
The number needed to treat with Georgium compared with placebo = 1/ARR = 1/0.5 = 2.

In this small trial the fictional drug, Georgium, would appear to be much better than placebo at achieving a 50% reduction in pain: only two patients would need to be treated to achieve a 50% reduction in pain.

6a. T
6b. T
6c. T
6d. T
It might reasonably be expected that you are aware of some of the commonly used statistical tests, although you would not be required to know how they might be applied.

7a. F
7b. F
7c. F
7d. F

Jasarch	Sarcoid	
	Present	**Absent**
Positive	$a=70$	$b=130$
Negative	$c=30$	$d=120$

Sensitivity $= a/(a+c) = 70/100 = 70\%$
Specificity $= d/(b+d) = 120/250 = 48\%$
Positive predictive value $= a/(a+b) = 70/200 = 35\%$
Negative predictive value $= d/(c+d) = 120/150 = 80\%$.

On the basis of these results it is unlikely that Jasarch would be adopted as a diagnostic test for sarcoid!

8a. F
8b. T
8c. T
8d. T
Likelihood ratios are powerful tools for assessing diagnostic accuracy of a test and are more clinically applicable than many other statistics. They are a clinical application of Bayes' theorem (first described by Rev. Thomas Bayes in 1763). They are calculated using the sensitivity and specificity of a test:

Positive likelihood ratio (LR+) $=$ sensitivity/($1-$specificity)
Negative likelihood ratio (LR−) $=$ ($1-$sensitivity)/specificity

A likelihood ratio >1 indicates that the test result is associated with disease and <1 that the test result is associated with absence of disease. A likelihood ratio of 1 indicates that the test is of no clinical utility. However, it is not until LR+ is >5 and LR− is <0.2 that they become most useful. The likelihood ratios can be applied to a pre-test probability (most easily using a nomogram) to estimate the post-test probability.

9a. T
9b. T
9c. T
9d. T
A trial can use a sample only to try to reflect the whole population being studied. Confidence intervals help us tell how much certainty there is around the result obtained in a trial. The narrower the confidence interval the more certain we can be that the trial result is precise. Confidence intervals are usually expressed as 95% or approximately 2 standard deviations either side of the trial result. They are useful only in parametric (normally distributed) data.

10a. T
10b. T
10c. T
10d. T
Type 1 and type 2 errors

	True state of the null hypothesis (H_0)	
Statistical decision	**True**	**False**
Reject H_0	Type 1 error	Correct
Do not reject H_0	Correct	Type 2 error

Type 1 errors (α, or false positive) occur when a true null hypothesis is incorrectly rejected. Type 2 errors (β, or false negative) occur when there is a failure to reject the null hypothesis when it is false. Type 1 errors are generally considered more serious than type 2 errors because they result in the null hypothesis being rejected when it is, in fact, true, whereas type 2 errors merely result in the null hypothesis not being rejected and no conclusion is drawn from the results. The probability of a type 1 error is set by the investigators (usually at a 5% level). The larger a sample size the closer the results will be to those for the whole population, so increasing the sample size will reduce both type 1 and type 2 errors. The power of a study is defined as $1 - \beta$.

10. Mock examination 1: Questions

1. Regarding pituitary hormones
a. Antidiuretic hormone (ADH) is secreted in response to a fall in serum osmolality
b. Dopamine stimulates the excretion of growth hormone
c. They all exert their effects via hormone release from target organs
d. ADH stimulates the release of adrenocorticotrophic hormone (ACTH)

2. Anatomical snuffbox
a. The anterior boundary is formed by the tendon of abductor pollicis longus and extensor pollicis brevis
b. The posterior boundary is formed by the tendon of extensor pollicis longus
c. The radial artery lies on the floor
d. Four bones can be palpated on the floor

3. Hypothalamic–thyroid axis
a. Both triiodothyronine (T_3) and thyroxine (T_4) induce a catabolic state
b. T_3 and T_4 act on receptors on the cell nucleus
c. Pituitary disease is suggested by a high thyroid-stimulating hormone (TSH), low T_3 and low T_4
d. Osteoporosis is a well-described complication of Graves' disease

4. Great saphenous vein
a. This arises on the dorsum of the foot
b. It travels posterior to the medial malleolus
c. It passes posterior to the lateral condyle of the femur
d. It drains into the femoral vein in the femoral triangle

5. Haemolytic uraemic syndrome (HUS)
a. This follows infection with *E. coli* or *Shigella* spp.
b. It occurs in most patients with bloody diarrhoea caused by *E. coli* O157
c. It is associated with thrombocytosis
d. It is a result of pathogen toxin production

6. **Amiodarone**
   a. This is useful in the treatment of both supraventricular and ventricular arrhythmias
   b. It slows phase 3 of the cardiac action potential and prolongs the refractory period in all cardiac tissues
   c. It is associated with serious endocrine, peripheral nervous system and pulmonary side effects
   d. It may decrease the serum level of warfarin

7. **Brachial plexus**
   a. This most commonly arises from the roots of C5–T1
   b. It has five roots, three trunks and three cords
   c. The cords are named based on their relationship to the brachial artery
   d. The roots pass anterior to the anterior scalene muscle in the neck

8. **Hip joint**
   a. This is a synovial ball-and-socket joint
   b. The femoral head receives its main blood supply from branches of the femoral artery via the ligamentum teres
   c. The ischiofemoral ligament prevents hyperflexion of the hip joint
   d. The femoral nerve supplies the hip joint

9. **Osmosis**
   a. This is the movement of solutes across a semipermeable membrane from areas of high concentration to areas of low concentration
   b. The osmotic pressure of a solution depends on the number of particles in solution
   c. If two fluids contain the same number of particles in a solution they exert the same osmotic pressure and are said to be 'isotonic'
   d. The osmolality is unaffected by temperature

10. **In patients with tuberculosis (TB)**
    a. Drug management of active TB is 6 months of isoniazid, rifampicin, pyrazinamide and ethambutol
    b. Patients with active, sputum-positive TB need to be barrier nursed at all times
    c. Multi-drug-resistant TB (MDR-TB) is more likely in HIV-infected individuals
    d. MDR-TB is more likely in patients residing in London

11. **Dermatomal innervation of the thoracic body wall**
    a. T4: level of the nipples
    b. T1: level of the clavicles
    c. T10: umbilicus
    d. The intercostal neurovascular bundles run on the superior aspect of the ribs

12. **Within the lung**
    a. Type I pneumocytes secrete surfactant
    b. Surfactant acts to increase surface tension, thereby preventing alveolar collapse
    c. A lack of surfactant contributes to the development of pulmonary oedema
    d. Smoking increases mucus and surfactant production

13. **Electrical activity of the heart**
    a. The cardiac cycle is initiated at the atrioventricular node
    b. The action potentials of cardiac muscle and skeletal muscle are similar
    c. The action potential of the cardiac pacemaker relies on the activation of fast Na^+ channels via gap junctions
    d. The action potential lasts almost as long as the cardiac cycle

14. **Inguinal canal**
    a. The roof of the inguinal canal is formed by the external oblique muscle
    b. The superficial ring lies inferior and medial to the pubic tubercle
    c. The deep ring lies approximately 1.25 cm superior to the middle of the inguinal ligament and lateral to the inferior epigastric artery
    d. The main occupant of the inguinal canal is the spermatic cord in males and the round ligament in females

15. **In the treatment of acute severe asthma**
    a. First-line drugs include the β-adrenoreceptor stimulants, muscarinic antagonists and xanthines
    b. Intravenous hydrocortisone is more effective than oral prednisolone
    c. Nebulised β_2 agonists can cause arterial hypoxaemia and should therefore be given with oxygen
    d. The dose of salbutamol when nebulised is 500 micrograms

16. **Jugular venous pulse**
    a. This reflects the right atrial pressure
    b. It changes throughout the cardiac cycle as pressure changes within the heart are transmitted from the left ventricle into the superior vena cava
    c. It has a 'c' wave that coincides with the contraction of the atria
    d. It has a 'v' wave that coincides with the contraction of the ventricles

17. **In the neck**
    a. There are three layers of deep cervical fascia in the neck
    b. There are four main tissue spaces in the neck
    c. Ludwig's angina is an infection of the retropharyngeal space
    d. Sternocleidomastoid muscle is supplied by the spinal accessory nerve

18. Peptic ulceration
   a. This predominantly occurs in the duodenum
   b. Occurring after major trauma or burns, it is known as Zollinger–Ellison syndrome
   c. It is usually associated with *Helicobacter pylori* infection
   d. It may be treated by reducing acid secretion with the use of H_1-receptor histamine antagonists such as ranitidine

19. Concerning liver biochemistry
   a. Raised serum aspartate transaminase (AST) reflects hepatocellular damage
   b. Cholestasis is indicated by raised γ-glutamyl transpeptidase (γGT)
   c. Serum bilirubin is usually in the conjugated form
   d. AST is specific to the liver

20. Stroke volume
   a. This is usually the same from both the left and the right ventricles
   b. It is equal to the end-systolic volume
   c. It is approximately 70 mL in the resting adult
   d. It may increase to 190 mL in endurance athletes

21. Regarding ocular palsies
   a. Lesions of the abducens (VI) nerve result in diplopia when looking down
   b. Lesions of the oculomotor (III) nerve result in the affected eye looking down and out
   c. Lesions of the trochlear (IV) nerve result in diplopia when looking towards the affected side
   d. An aneurysm of the posterior cerebral or superior cerebellar artery can cause a complete oculomotor (III) nerve palsy

22. Proton pump inhibitors (PPIs)
   a. The H^+/K^+ ATPase (proton pump) is located on the parietal cell and catalyses the exchange of extracellular H^+ for intracellular K^+
   b. PPIs bind irreversibly to the stimulated proton pumps
   c. It is best to take PPIs before the first meal of the day for maximal effect
   d. Side effects such as abdominal pain, diarrhoea and constipation are rare

23. Atlas (first cervical vertebra) and axis (second cervical vertebra)
   a. The atlas has no vertebral body
   b. The transverse ligament prevents vertical displacement of the atlas on the axis
   c. A hangman's fracture is a fracture through the odontoid peg
   d. The axis has a bifid spinous process

24. Wound healing
a. Mucous membrane healing is more efficient than that of skin
b. The liver demonstrates complete and rapid regeneration
c. Nerve cells in the peripheral nervous system will regenerate
d. Contact inhibition is a process used to control wound healing

25. In Advanced Life Support of patients in cardiac arrest
a. The dose of adrenaline (epinephrine) is 10 mL of 1:1000
b. Amiodarone may be useful after the fourth cycle of CPR in the treatment of pulseless electrical activity (PEA)
c. Atropine is indicated in patients with asystole or PEA with a rate <60/min
d. Adrenaline should be given just after the delivery of the first shock

26. Glomerular filtration rate (GFR)
a. This is approximately 180 litres/day
b. Up to 50% of the total amount of fluid filtered is returned to the circulation by tubular reabsorption
c. It can be estimated after an infusion of insulin
d. It may increase if the plasma protein concentration is low

27. After an episode of trauma the following metabolic changes occur in the human stress response
a. The urine is likely to be more concentrated
b. Aldosterone secretion is decreased
c. Cytokine production is increased
d. Interleukin-6 promotes the acute phase response

28. The following statements about the anion gap are true
a. Routine serum analysis measures more anions than cations
b. The anion gap is usually 25–30 mmol/L
c. Most states of acidosis have a normal anion gap value
d. Renal tubular acidosis may have a normal anion gap

29. Regarding hyperprolactinaemia
a. Only women are affected
b. It may occur naturally during sleep
c. It may present with osteoporosis
d. It may occur in a patient on metoclopramide

30. Concerning the innate immune system
a. Previous exposure to the pathogen is required for a response
b. It acts as the first line of defence
c. It requires B lymphocytes
d. It involves macrophages and neutrophils

31. **The following conditions result in abnormally coloured urine**
    a. Rhabdomyolysis
    b. Congenital porphyria
    c. Treatment with rifampicin
    d. Phenylketonuria

32. **Iron deficiency anaemia**
    a. Postmenopausal women are the most commonly affected group of patients
    b. It may be caused by coeliac disease
    c. The total iron-binding capacity (TIBC) is low
    d. The blood film is likely to show hypochromia

33. **Medial compartment of the thigh**
    a. This contains the adductor muscles
    b. It is supplied by the femoral nerve
    c. It contains the adductor canal
    d. The muscles of the medial compartment adduct and medially rotate the leg

34. **Factor V Leiden deficiency**
    a. This is an autosomal recessive inherited disorder resulting in reduced factor V levels
    b. Presentation is often with bleeding gums
    c. The bleeding time is usually increased
    d. Bleeding usually requires treatment with vitamin K

35. **Functional residual capacity**
    a. This is increased in obese individuals
    b. It is higher in males than females
    c. It increases on standing from a lying position
    d. It increases during general anaesthesia

36. **In cases of cellulitis**
    a. Antibiotic treatment should cover Gram-negative organisms
    b. The affected area is usually tender
    c. When it affects the foot, treatment for athlete's foot is advised if present
    d. The affected area of the body should be rested

37. **Thiazide diuretics**
    a. These act mainly on the early segments of the proximal tubule
    b. They may cause hypokalaemia and metabolic acidosis
    c. They should be used with caution in patients with diabetes
    d. They are secreted by the same system that secretes uric acid and may precipitate gout

38. **Regarding potential errors in a study**
    a. A type 1 error (α) is the incorrect rejection of the null hypothesis when it is true
    b. The probability of a type 1 error is the same as the significance level
    c. Assuming that all other conditions stay the same, increasing the sample size will always reduce the chance of both type 1 and type 2 errors
    d. If the sample size stays the same, reducing the chance of a type 1 error will increase the chance of a type 2 error

39. **Calcaneal fractures**
    a. These are usually caused by eversion injuries
    b. They are usually associated with an increase in Bohler's angle
    c. They are associated with fractures around the pelvis
    d. If they are recognised and treated, complete recovery is the rule

40. **Intravenous fluids**
    a. Physiological (0.9%) saline has the same similar sodium concentration as extracellular fluid
    b. Maintenance fluids for an 8-year-old of average weight would be 1580 mL/day
    c. For a patient with burns, maximum fluid requirement can be calculated using Parkland's formula
    d. A patient with burns should receive fluid 10 mL/kg per % BSA, over 24 hours

41. **A prolonged prothrombin time is seen in the following**
    a. Vitamin K deficiency
    b. Liver failure
    c. Heparin use
    d. Factor VIII deficiency

42. **Herpes simplex**
    a. Herpes simplex causing genital lesions is usually due to HSV-2
    b. It is an RNA virus
    c. Primary infection may be asymptomatic
    d. Secondary reactivation results in shingles

43. **In acute lymphoblastic leukaemia**
    a. There is malignant transformation of the lymphocyte
    b. Presentation is often with signs of bone marrow failure
    c. Cure rates of up to 80% in children have been described
    d. Poor prognosis is associated with mediastinal disease at presentation

44. **Causes of ST-segment elevation on an ECG include the following**
    a. Prinzmetal's angina
    b. Subarachnoid haemorrhage
    c. Ventricular aneurysm
    d. Digoxin

45. **After envenomation by the European adder, the following are indications for the administration of antivenom**
    a. Persistent hypotension
    b. A white cell count $>20 \times 10^9$/L
    c. Massive limb swelling
    d. A raised lactate dehydrogenase (LDH)

46. **When describing the results of a trial of a diagnostic test**
    a. The sensitivity is the proportion of people with the disease who have a positive test
    b. The negative predictive value decreases with increasing prevalence
    c. A positive test in the presence of a high specificity can help rule in the disease
    d. The positive predictive value indicates how likely a patient who tests positive is to have the disease

47. **The following statements about haemolytic anaemias are true**
    a. Patients may present with gallstones
    b. In glucose-6-phosphate dehydrogenase deficiency, ingestion of fava beans may lead to anaemia and jaundice
    c. Infection is a common trigger for haemolysis
    d. Hereditary spherocytosis is an X-linked disorder

48. **The following are examples of fungal infections**
    a. Aspergillosis
    b. Brucellosis
    c. *Pneumocystis jirovecii* (formerly *P. carinii*) pneumonia
    d. Hydatid disease

49. **Regarding the thrombin time**
    a. A normal range is 10–15 seconds
    b. It will be increased in patients with vitamin K deficiency
    c. It is raised in patients receiving heparin
    d. It is raised in haemophilia A

50. *Escherichia coli*
    a. Enterotoxigenic strains are the most common cause of travellers' diarrhoea
    b. It is an anaerobic bacterium
    c. It is a Gram-positive organism
    d. Infection may cause the haemolytic uraemic syndrome

10. Mock examination 1: Answers

1a. F
1b. F
1c. F
1d. T

ADH is secreted from the posterior lobe of the pituitary in response to an increase in plasma osmolality or a decrease in blood pressure. ADH acts to increase water absorption from the renal collecting tubules/ducts in response to rises in extracellular fluid osmolality, as detected by hypothalamic osmoreceptors. ADH stimulates the release of ACTH, in synergy with corticotrophin-releasing hormone (CRH). Dopamine increases the excretion of prolactin, which is the only pituitary hormone that does not act via a target endocrine gland.

2a. T
2b. T
2c. T
2d. T

The four bones that can be palpated on the floor of the anatomical snuffbox are, from proximal to distal, the radial styloid, scaphoid, trapezium and base of the first metacarpal.

3a. T
3b. T
3c. F
3d. T

T_3 and T_4 act to induce metabolism and are essential for growth and mental development. Both T_3 and T_4 act on nuclear receptors to induce catabolism. A high TSH, low T_3 and low T_4 suggest thyroid disease, i.e. hypothyroidism. Pituitary disease would be suggested by all the tests being low. Graves' disease is likely to produce ophthalmoplegia, congestive cardiac failure, atrial fibrillation, osteoporosis and gynaecomastia, in addition to the usual signs of hyperthyroidism.

4a. T
4b. F
4c. F
4d. T

The great saphenous vein is formed by the union of the dorsal vein of the great toe and the dorsal venous arch of the foot. It passes anterior to the medial malleolus and posterior to the medial condyle of the femur. It drains into the femoral vein in the femoral triangle.

5a. T
5b. F
5c. F
5d. T
HUS occurs in 5–10% of infections with *E. coli* O157, but it may also follow streptococcal, Coxsackievirus, echovirus and adenovirus infection. HUS is characterised by a microangiopathic haemolytic anaemia, acute renal failure and thrombocytopenia.

6a. T
6b. T
6c. T
6d. F
Amiodarone blocks several different ion channels, including K^+ and inactivated Na^+ channels, as well as β-adrenoreceptors. Although useful in the treatment of both supraventricular and ventricular arrhythmias, it may cause serious side effects and, because of this, its use for maintenance should be limited to when other agents have failed. It causes an increase in the serum level of many drugs including warfarin and digoxin.

7a. T
7b. T
7c. F
7d. F
The brachial plexus commonly arises from C5–T1; sometimes there is a small contribution from C4 or T2. The cords are named based on their relationship to the axillary artery. The roots of the brachial plexus usually pass through the gap between the anterior and middle scalene muscle, along with the subclavian artery.

8a. T
8b. F
8c. F
8d. T
The femoral head receives its main blood supply from the femoral artery but via the lateral and medial circumflex arteries, which pass to the head by running along the femoral neck. There is a small artery to the head that passes through the ligamentum teres but this arises from the obturator artery. The hip joint is strengthened by ligaments. The Y-shaped iliofemoral ligament reinforces the capsule anteriorly and prevents hyperextension of the joint. The capsule is reinforced on the inferior and anterior aspects by the pubofemoral ligament. This ligament prevents hyperabduction of the hip joint. The ischiofemoral ligament reinforces the posterior aspect and prevents hyperextension. The hip joint receives innervation from the femoral nerve, obturator nerve, superior gluteal nerve, nerve to quadratus femoris and accessory obturator nerve (if present).

9a. F
9b. T
9c. T
9d. T
Osmosis is the passive movement of water across a semipermeable membrane from areas of low solute concentration to areas of high concentration. Fluids with the same number of particles are isotonic; those with a higher number of solutes are hypertonic and those with a lower number of solute hypotonic. Osmolarity (osmol/L) is the concentration of all osmotically active particles in a solution regardless of the compounds or mixtures involved. Osmolality is a measure of osmoles of solute per kilogram of solvent. As temperature affects volume of water, this will have an effect on osmolarity, but not osmolality, and hence osmolality is the measurement favoured by physiologists.

10a. F
10b. F
10c. T
10d. T
TB treatment generally consists of an initial three- or four-drug phase followed by a 4-month continuation phase – typically 6 months of isoniazid and rifampicin with an initial 2 months of additional ethambutol and pyrazinamide. The patient should wear a mask when leaving his or her room; respiratory isolation is essential in the presence of HIV-positive patients. MDR-TB should be suspected in patients with prior TB treatment; known contact with MDR-TB; HIV-positive individuals; age 25–44; males; and those residing in London or born overseas.

11a. T
11b. F
11c. T
11d. F
The T1 dermatome lies on the inner aspect of upper arms. The intercostal neurovascular bundle runs in the costal groove on the inferior aspect of each rib so, when performing thoracocentesis, one must ensure that the needle is inserted just superiorly to a rib, to prevent damage to the neurovascular bundle.

12a. F
12b. F
12c. T
12d. F
Type II pneumocytes secrete the phospholipid–protein complex surfactant, which reduces surface tension to prevent alveolar collapse. Smoking increases mucus production but decreases surfactant production.

13a. F
13b. F
13c. F
13d. T
The sinoatrial (SA) node is the site of initiation of the cardiac cycle via specialised cells that slowly depolarise after every action potential. This is dependent on a slow influx of calcium ions (Ca^{2+}). The action potential of cardiac muscle differs significantly from skeletal muscle. To prevent any chance of tetany, the refractory period of the cardiac action potential lasts until just before the next depolarisation.

14a. F
14b. F
14c. T
14d. T
The anterior wall of the inguinal canal is formed by the aponeurosis of the external oblique muscle (EOM) and is reinforced laterally by the internal oblique muscle (IOM). The posterior wall is formed by transversalis fascia with the medial part being reinforced by the conjoint tendon of the IOM and the transversalis abdominis muscle (TAM). The roof is formed by the arching fibres of IOM and TAM, and the floor by the in-curving of the inguinal ligament, which is reinforced medially by the lacunar ligament. The superficial ring is a slit-like opening between the fibres of the aponeurosis of the EOM, and lies superior and lateral to the pubic tubercle. The deep ring is formed by an outpouching of transversalis fascia.

15a. F
15b. F
15c. T
15d. F
First-line treatment in acute severe asthma includes β-adrenoreceptor stimulants such as salbutamol and muscarinic antagonists such as ipratropium. Xanthines such as theophylline may be used as part of the treatment strategy, but only if other agents are not providing adequate relief. The action of both prednisolone and hydrocortisone is similar with no temporal advantage of the intravenous over the oral preparation. The dose of nebulised salbutamol is 5 mg, and that of ipratropium 500 micrograms.

16a. T
16b. F
16c. F
16d. F
The jugular venous pulse can be a valuable tool in the cardiovascular examination. It directly reflects the right atrial pressure because there are no valves between the right atrium and the jugular vein. The different waves seen in the jugular venous pulse relate to the following parts of the cardiac cycle: 'a' wave – atrial systole; 'c' wave – bulging of the atrioventricular (AV) valves into the atria as right ventricular pressure increases; 'v' wave – closure of the tricuspid valve and atrial filling.

17a. F
17b. T
17c. F
17d. T

There are four layers of deep cervical fascia in the neck: the investing layer, pretracheal fascia, prevertebral fascia and carotid sheath. There are four main tissue spaces:

1. Submandibular space: the investing fascia splits to enclose the submandibular gland and the mylohyoid muscle.
2. Retropharyngeal space: lies immediately anterior to the prevertebral fascia and extends distally behind the oesophagus to the diaphragm via the superior and then posterior mediastinum. This connection allows infection to spread easily into the mediastinum.
3. Prevertebral space is behind the prevertebral fascia. This space allows infection to track down into the axilla via the axillary sheath.
4. The parapharyngeal space lies between the thyroid and the buccopharyngeal fascia.

Ludwig's angina is an infection of the submandibular space often secondary to a dental infection. Swelling can cause the tongue to be displaced backwards, resulting in airway obstruction.

18a. T
18b. F
18c. T
18d. F

Duodenal ulceration is two to three times more common than gastric ulcer. Curling's ulcer occurs after trauma/stress. Zollinger–Ellison syndrome is a gastrin-secreting pancreatic adenoma, leading to excess acid secretion. *Helicobacter pylori* infection is associated with 95% of duodenal and 80% of gastric ulcers. H_2-receptor histamine antagonists such as ranitidine reduce acid secretion.

19a. T
19b. T
19c. F
19d. F

Transaminases or aminotransferases are present in hepatocytes, which leak into the blood when liver cell damage is present. AST is a mitochondrial enzyme, found in cardiac, muscle, renal, brain and hepatic tissue. ALT (alanine transaminase) is a cytosol enzyme and is more specific to the liver. Cholestasis produces a rise in alkaline phosphatase (ALP) and γGT. Circulating bilirubin is normally almost all unconjugated.

20a. T
20b. F
20c. T
20d. T
The ventricle output of the left and right systems must be balanced and equal. If the stroke volume from the right ventricle were to be greater than that of the left, blood would accumulate in the pulmonary system, with resulting fluid being pushed into the lung (pulmonary oedema). The stroke volume is equal to the end-systolic volume minus the end-diastolic volume (ESV − EDV). Even at maximal exertion the heart is unable to empty fully. The usual 'ejection fraction' is approximately 60%.

21a. F
21b. T
21c. F
21d. T
The superior oblique muscle turns the eyeball inferiorly and medially. Lesions of the trochlear nerve result in diplopia on looking down, i.e. walking down the stairs. With an oculomotor nerve palsy, only the superior oblique and lateral rectus muscles continue to function, so the eyeball is pulled laterally and inferiorly (down and out). A complete lesion of the oculomotor nerve results in both the motor and parasympathetic components being affected, causing ptosis, no pupillary light reflex, dilatation of the pupil, no accommodation response, and an eye that looks down and out. Complete lesions are caused by external compression of the third nerve, e.g. by a posterior cerebral artery aneurysm. In a partial oculomotor nerve palsy, only the motor component is affected. This is because these lesions are caused by processes that directly affect the nerve fibres, e.g. diabetes, and, as the parasympathetic fibres run along the outside of the nerve, they are unaffected in partial lesions. The abducens nerve nucleus lies in the pons. The abducens nerve supplies the lateral rectus muscle, so the affected eye is unable to abduct, resulting in diplopia when looking towards the side of the lesion.

22a. F
22b. T
22c. T
22d. F
The H^+/K^+ ATPase (proton pump) is located on the apical portion of the parietal cell and increases the amount of acid in the gastric secretions via the exchange of intracellular H^+ and extracellular K^+. As the number of proton pumps is maximised in the fasting state the proton pump inhibitors should be given first thing in the morning before eating. Gastrointestinal side effects are common.

23a. T
23b. F
23c. F
23d. T
The first cervical vertebra (the atlas) is a ring-shaped bone. The superior articular surface receives the two occipital condyles. The atlas has no spinous

process or body; it consists of an anterior and posterior arch, each of which has a tubercle and a lateral mass. The second cervical vertebra (axis) has two large, flat, weight-bearing surfaces on which the atlas rotates. The axis has an odontoid process (peg), which projects superiorly from its body. The odontoid process is held in position by the transverse ligament, which prevents horizontal displacement. The axis has a large bifid spinous process. A hangman's fracture is a fracture through the pedicles of the axis.

24a. T
24b. T
24c. T
24d. T
The skin has limited powers of regeneration and mucous membrane healing is more efficient. Wounds in the mouth rarely need suturing. The liver shows complete regeneration and healing. Nerve cells do not divide and cannot be replaced. However, injured cells in the peripheral system will regenerate and axoplasm can push into an endoneural tube at 2–3 mm/day.
Contact inhibition is a process where contact between cells of the same type suppresses division and motility. The apposed cells form junctions allowing intracellular signals to flow from cell to cell.

25a. F
25b. F
25c. T
25d. F
The dose of adrenaline (epinephrine) in cardiac arrest is 1 mg, which is 10 mL of 1:10 000, and consensus opinion from the Resuscitation Council is that it should be given just before the third shock. Amiodarone may be useful in the treatment of persistent ventricular fibrillation/tachycardia (VF/VT).

26a. T
26b. F
26c. F
26d. T
The GFR is the total volume of fluid filtered by the glomeruli per unit time. It is normally about 120 mL/min per 1.73 m^2 of body surface area (BSA about 180 L/day). Clearly most of this must be reabsorbed to maintain the circulating volume and about 99% of the GFR returns to the extracellular compartment via tubular reabsorption. GFR can be measured using inulin (not insulin), which is freely filterable, is not metabolised by the kidney and does not alter renal function, and the filtered amount does not change as a result of reabsorption or secretion in the tubule. If the plasma protein concentration is low, this will reduce oncotic pressure and therefore increase GFR.

27a. T
27b. F
27c. T
27d. T
The stress response is the name given to a set of hormonal, neuroendocrine and metabolic changes that follow surgery and trauma. Generally there

is increased secretion of pituitary hormones, which promotes a state of catabolism that mobilises substrates to provide energy for the body to recover. Essentially these include:

- Increased ACTH and growth hormone (GH) secretion (promotes a catabolic state and causes insulin resistance)
- Decreased thyroxine secretion
- Increased vasopressin secretion
- Increased cortisol and aldosterone
- Decreased insulin secretion
- Increased glucagon secretion
- Increased cytokine production (IL-6, tumour necrosis factor [TNF])
- Neutrophil leukocytosis
- Lymphocyte proliferation.

These all lead to a catabolic state so breakdown of fat and protein and glycogen is promoted, as is the production of glucose.

28a. F
28b. F
28c. F
28d. T
Routine serum analysis measures more cations (Na^+ and K^+) than anions (Cl^- and HCO_3^-). The difference is referred to as the anion gap and is usually in the range of 10–16 mmol/L, reflecting the presence of unmeasured anions. Most states of acidosis will have a raised anion gap (lactic acidosis, renal failure, ketosis, alcohol, diabetes, salicylate poisoning). A normal anion gap may be present in renal tubular acidosis, diarrhoea, acetazolamide poisoning, Addison's disease and ammonium chloride ingestion.

29a. F
29b. T
29c. T
29d. T
Hyperprolactinaemia is the most common pituitary abnormality. It is usually caused by a prolactin-secreting anterior pituitary adenoma. It tends to present early in women (amenorrhoea/galactorrhoea) and late in men (loss of libido and facial hair). It may also present with osteoporosis. Physiological hyper-prolactinaemia occurs in breastfeeding, sleep and pregnancy, but may also be secondary to dopamine antagonist because dopamine is the hypothalamic stimulant for prolactin secretion.

30a. F
30b. T
30c. F
30d. T
The adaptive immune system requires previous pathogen exposure. B- and T-cell clones respond to specific antigens as part of the response. The innate system provides the initial, non-specific response to pathogens, and most leukocytes, except B lymphocytes, are involved.

31a. T
31b. T
31c. T
31d. F
Rhabdomyolysis results in myoglobin in the urine, which often shows as a darker-coloured urine. Porphyria results in porphyrinogens in the urine, which are colourless but become dark red on contact with light. Rifampicin stains most body fluids pink.

32a. F
32b. T
32c. F
32d. T
In the Western world the most common cause of iron deficiency is menstruation. Malabsorption as a result of small bowel disease or hookworm infestation is another well-documented cause. Iron deficiency results in microcytosis and hypochromia on a blood film. The MCV (mean corpuscular volume) is low, as are the total iron and transferrin. The binding capacity will therefore be high. Below is a comparison of iron, TIBC and transferrin states in various anaemias:

Type of anaemia	Iron	TIBC	Transferrin
Iron deficiency	↓	↑	↓
Anaemia of chronic disease	↓	↓	↑
Chronic haemolysis	↑	↓	↑
Haemochromatosis	↑	↓	↑
Sideroblastic anaemia	↑	↔	↑

33a. T
33b. F
33c. T
33d. T
The medial compartment of the upper leg contains adductor longus, adductor magnus, adductor brevis, gracilis and obturator externus. The obturator nerve supplies them all (L2, L3, L4) except for the hamstring part of adductor magnus, which is supplied by the tibial branch of the sciatic nerve. The adductor canal is an opening in the aponeurotic distal attachment of adductor magnus. The adductor canal transmits the femoral artery and vein from the anterior thigh to the popliteal fossa. The muscles of the medial compartment adduct and medially rotate the leg.

34a. T
34b. T
34c. F
34d. F
Also known as Owren's disease, factor V deficiency is a rare autosomal recessive condition leading to reduced factor V levels. Presentation is commonly with bleeding (gums, skin, joints) and is usually treated with fresh frozen plasma. The aPPT (activated partial prothrombin time) is increased but the bleeding time is usually normal.

35a. F
35b. T
35c. T
35d. F
Functional residual capacity (FRC), a combination of expiratory reserve volume and residual volume, is decreased in pregnancy, obesity, supine position and anaesthesia. The application of PEEP (positive end-expiratory pressure) increases FRC.

36a. F
36b. T
36c. T
36d. T
Cellulitis is a superficial skin infection. It is nearly always the result of either staphylococcal or streptococcal infection. Infection usually gets into the skin via a cut, insect bite or any break to the skin, e.g. athlete's foot (which should also be treated if present). The skin is red and tender, and may blister. Treatment is rest and elevation (lower limbs), and antibiotic treatment.

37a. F
37b. F
37c. T
37d. T
Thiazide diuretics include bendroflumethiazide, indapamide and metolazone. They act on the early segments of the distal tubule, increasing excretion of Cl^-, Na^+ and H_2O, by binding on the channel responsible for co-transport of Na^+/Cl^- and inhibiting NaCl reabsorption. As they increase excretion of K^+ and H^+, they cause hypokalaemia and metabolic alkalosis. They impair glucose tolerance and secretion of uric acid.

38a. T
38b. T
38c. T
38d. T
Type 1 and type 2 errors

	True state of the null hypothesis (H_0)	
Statistical decision	True	False
Reject H_0	Type 1 error	Correct
Do not reject H_0	Correct	Type 2 error

Type 1 errors (α, or false positive) occur when a true null hypothesis is incorrectly rejected. Type 2 errors (β, or false negative) occur when there is a failure to reject the null hypothesis when it is false. Type 1 errors are generally considered more serious than type 2 errors because they result in the null hypothesis being rejected when it is, in fact, true, whereas type 2 errors merely result in the null hypothesis not being rejected and no conclusion is drawn from the results. The probability of a type 1 error is set by the investigators (usually at a 5% level). The larger a sample size the closer the results will be to those for the whole population, so increasing the sample size will reduce both type 1 and type 2 errors. The power of a study is defined as $1 - \beta$.

39a. F
39b. F
39c. T
39d. F
Calcaneal fractures usually result from a fall from a height or axial loading, and are associated with severe trauma and pelvic and spinal fractures. Bohler's angle is the angle between a line connecting the superior aspects of the posterior facet and the superior aspect of the anterior process and a line drawn from the posterior facet to the calcaneal tuberosity. Normally the angle is approximately $25-40°$ but decreases in fractures of the calcaneum. Secondary osteoarthritis is very common following calcaneal fractures, especially when involving the subtalar joint.

40a. F
40b. T
40c. F
40d. F
Physiological (0.9%) saline contains 150 mmol/l sodium, so more than plasma (which contains 135–145 mmol/L). Daily maintenance fluid requirements for a child can be calculated as 100 mL/kg for the first 10 kg, 50 mL/kg for the second 10 kg, and 20 mL/kg for remaining kilograms. An average-sized 8-year-old weighs approximately 24 kg when estimated using the APLS (Advanced Paediatric Life Support) formula ([age + 4] × 2) so the maintenance fluid requirement for 24 hours would be 1000 mL (for the first 10 kg of body weight) + 500 mL (for the second 10 kg of body weight) + 80 mL (for the

remaining 4 kg of body weight) $=$ 1580 mL. Patients with burns require larger volumes of fluid and Parkland's formula is one formula used to calculate requirements (4 mL/kg per % BSA [body surface area] over 24 hours from time of burn); however, additional fluid may be needed, based on other measurements of volume status, e.g. urine output.

41a. T
41b. T
41c. F
41d. F
Prothrombin time (PT) is a measure of the extrinsic coagulation pathway function. This involves the hepatic-derived, vitamin K-dependent clotting factors II, V, VII and X, together with fibrinogen. Heparin binds and activates antithrombin, inactivating thrombin and factor Xa. It prolongs the activated partial thromboplastic time ratio (APTR), a measure of the intrinsic coagulation pathway.

42a. T
42b. F
42c. T
42d. F
Herpes simplex is a DNA virus. Although not rigid, subtypes of HSV-1 generally cause cold sores, herpetic stomatitis and encephalitis, whereas HSV-2 causes genital herpes (and occasionally pharyngitis and meningitis). Primary type I infection may go unnoticed – about 70% of the population are infected but only a third suffer recurrence in the form of cold sores. Varicella-zoster reactivation causes herpes zoster or shingles.

43a. F
43b. T
43c. T
43d. T
In all leukaemias there is malignant transformation of the lymphoblast which infiltrates the marrow (resulting in failure), and lymphoblasts are often seen on the peripheral blood film. It is the most common malignancy seen in children and is more common in boys. It peaks in incidence at 2–5 years. It often presents with anaemia, thrombocytopenia and leukopenia. Bone pain is common and in T-cell disease there is often a mediastinal mass seen on chest radiograph. The lymphoblasts stain negative for Sudan black and peroxidase, but stain positive with periodic acid–Schiff (PAS). Initial treatment to induce remission is chemotherapy with prednisolone and vincristine. Intrathecal methotrexate is also commonly used. Cure rates of up to 80% have been described.

Poor prognostic factors include:

- Counts $>$20 000 at presentation
- Age $<$2 or $>$10 years
- Males
- Those with an associated chromosomal defect
- T-cell disease.

44a. T
44b. T
44c. T
44d. F
There are many causes of ST-segment elevation on an ECG apart from myocardial infarction. These include Prinzmetal's angina (coronary vaso-spasm), ventricular aneurysm, left ventricular hypertrophy, pericarditis and hypertrophic cardiomyopathy. A large proportion of patients with significant subarachnoid haemorrhage have ST-segment elevation. Digoxin causes ST-segment depression, classically accompanied by a 'reverse tick' in the lateral leads.

45a. T
45b. T
45c. T
45d. F
Deaths from adder envenomation are rare – the last in the UK was in 1975. The European adder rarely bites, usually only as a last resort in response to extreme provocation. The following are indications for the administration of antivenom:

- Persistent (>2 hours) fall in blood pressure (systolic to <80 mmHg or a decrease of more than 50 mmHg from normal or admission value) with or without signs of shock
- Hypotension unresponsive to fluid therapy
- Definite leukocytosis (especially if >20 × 1 000 000 000/L)
- ECG abnormalities
- Acidosis
- Elevated creatine kinase
- Severe local envenomation within 4 hours of the bite (even in the absence of systemic signs), i.e. swelling beyond the next major joint from bite site (or more than half the bitten limb within 48 hours); any cases involving significant swelling of forearm or leg should also receive antivenom
- Any other evidence of systemic envenomation, e.g. pulmonary oedema, spontaneous bleeding.

46a. T
46b. T
46c. T
46d. T
The prevalence of a disease is the proportion of the population who have the disease. Sensitivity and specificity are unaffected by the prevalence of a disease, whereas positive and negative predictive values will change depending on the prevalence. A negative test in the presence of a high sensitivity will help rule out the disease ('SnOUT') and a positive test in the presence of a high sensitivity will help rule in the diagnosis ('SpIN').

47a. T
47b. T
47c. T
47d. F
Haemolysis is the premature destruction of erythrocytes, and leads to haemolytic anaemia when bone marrow activity cannot compensate for the erythrocyte loss.

There are many causes. G6PDH (glucose-6-phosphate dehydrogenase) deficiency is an X-linked disorder where haemolysis is precipitated by oxidative drugs, e.g. sulphonamides or ciprofloxacin, ingestion of fava beans or infection. Hereditary spherocytosis is an autosomal dominant condition leading to osmotic fragility of the abnormal red cell membrane. Splenomegaly is common. Often the haemolysis can be autoimmune or secondary to drugs or infection. Haemolysis can lead to anaemia, jaundice and haemosiderin gallstones.

48a. T
48b. F
48c. T
48d. F
Aspergillosis results from infection with the fungus *Aspergillus*. It usually affects the lungs of susceptible individuals, e.g. immunocompromised patients. Brucellosis is a condition caused by Gram-negative rods. It is associated with ingestion of unpasteurised milk. *Pneumocystis* sp. was originally thought to be protozoan but has been reclassified as a fungal infection. It mainly affects the lungs of those with AIDS. Hydatid disease is the result of a tapeworm infestation.

49a. T
49b. F
49c. T
49d. F
Thrombin is added to plasma to convert fibrinogen to fibrin. The thrombin time (10–15 s) is increased in heparin therapy, disseminated intravascular coagulation (DIC) and afibrinogenaemia.

50a. T
50b. F
50c. F
50d. T
Escherichia coli is an aerobic, Gram-negative organism. It commonly causes urinary tract infections, bacteraemia and neonatal meningitis. It is the most common cause of travellers' diarrhoea. *E. coli* O157:H7 infection is associated with the development of haemolytic uraemic syndrome, particularly in children.

11. Mock examination 2: Questions

1. The femoral sheath
a. This is formed by the inferior prolongation of tranversalis and iliopsoas fascia
b. It encloses the femoral nerve, artery and vein
c. It has two compartments
d. It contains the femoral canal at the medial aspect

2. Cortisol
a. Most of the circulating cortisol is bound to albumin
b. Secretion of cortisol follows a circadian rhythm, peaking at midnight
c. It is secreted from the zona fasciculata of the adrenal glands
d. Secretion is increased by emotional stress

3. The following are correct virus and disease pairings
a. Herpes simplex – chickenpox
b. CMV – glandular fever
c. Parvovirus – slapped-cheek syndrome
d. Paromyxovirus – measles

4. Blood supply of the lower limb
a. The femoral artery arises from the internal iliac artery
b. The femoral artery has no branches
c. The femoral artery divides into the anterior and posterior tibial arteries
d. The dorsalis pedis artery arises from the posterior tibial artery

5. Acute myeloid leukaemia (AML)
a. Patients may present with bleeding and purpura
b. Intrathecal (IT) methotrexate is commonly given
c. Patients may present with features of DIC
d. Bone marrow transplantation therapy may be indicated in younger patients

6. In hyperparathyroidism the following statements are true
a. Increased parathyroid hormone is usually a result of a malignant adenoma
b. It may present with polydipsia
c. The serum calcium is often raised in secondary hyperparathyroidism
d. It is often associated with radiographic evidence of bone resorption

7. **Avascular necrosis is commonly seen in the following**
   a. Scaphoid fractures
   b. Fractures of the lunate
   c. Colles' fractures
   d. Femoral shaft fractures

8. **Blood film analysis**
   a. Hypochromia may be seen in the blood film of patients with thalassaemia
   b. Basophilic stippling is pathognomonic of lead poisoning
   c. Blast cells may be a normal finding
   d. Poikilocytes are associated with iron deficiency anaemia

9. **Likelihood ratios**
   a. A likelihood ratio is calculated using the positive and negative predictive values
   b. A positive likelihood ratio >10 strongly rules in the disease being tested for
   c. A negative likelihood ratio <0.1 strongly rules out the disease being tested for
   d. Likelihood ratios are useful only when applied to the post-test probability

10. **Cushing's syndrome**
    a. Its main effects are secondary to raised aldosterone levels
    b. The most common endogenous cause is a pituitary tumour
    c. It is associated with ectopic ACTH secretion from a bronchial adenocarcinoma
    d. It is associated with osteoporosis

11. **Flecainide**
    a. This is effective for controlling both supraventricular and ventricular arrhythmias
    b. It acts on potassium channels and slows repolarisation
    c. It can be given safely to patients with poor myocardial function
    d. It has a negative inotropic action

12. **The scalp**
    a. This has six layers
    b. Scalp lacerations very rarely bleed
    c. The arterial supply to the scalp runs in the subaponeurotic space (layer 4)
    d. Scalp infections do not spread intracranially

13. Heparin
a. Low-molecular-weight heparins are preferable to intravenous heparin because regular monitoring of the aPTT is usually not required
b. Low-molecular-weight heparins do not cause thrombocytopenia
c. It should be avoided in patients taking angiotensin II receptor antagonists
d. It may cause priapism in men

14. Pleura
a. The parietal pleura is innervated by the intercostals and phrenic nerves
b. The visceral pleura is innervated by the autonomic nervous system
c. The pleura covering the apex of the lung never extends above the level of the second rib
d. The parietal pleura is insensitive to pain

15. Carbon dioxide is transported in blood
a. Bound to haemoglobin as carboxyhaemoglobin
b. Mostly as bicarbonate
c. More readily in oxygenated blood according to the Haldane effect
d. In red blood cells more than in plasma

16. Regarding the sinoatrial node
a. Its action potential is the same as that of ventricular muscle
b. The resting potential is greater than that of ventricular muscle
c. Its action potential is created by the influx of sodium ions through fast Na^+ channels
d. It is blocked by the administration of adenosine

17. Saliva
a. Primary secretion from the acini is an isotonic fluid
b. Sympathetic stimulation is blocked by atropine
c. It contains amylase, ribonuclease and lipase
d. Secretion is controlled via nuclei in the hypothalamus

18. Thoracic inlet
a. The oesophagus lies posterior to the trachea
b. The aortic arch gives rise directly to the left and right subclavian arteries, and the left and right common carotid arteries
c. The left brachiocephalic vein crosses posterior to the left common carotid artery to enter the superior vena cava
d. The trachea lies posterior to all the major blood vessels at the thoracic inlet

19. *Campylobacter*
    a. Infection is usually via contaminated seafood
    b. It causes bloody diarrhoea
    c. It is associated with headache and myalgia
    d. It may result in a reactive arthritis

20. The stomach
    a. This is divided into four regions
    b. It is supplied by the gastric arteries that arise from the superior mesenteric artery
    c. It receives its sympathetic nerve supply via the vagus nerve
    d. It lies anterior to the pancreas

21. Concerning the ventilation–perfusion ratio ($\dot{V}/\dot{Q}$)
    a. In the upright position ventilation is maximal at the lung base
    b. In the upright position perfusion is maximal at the apices of the lung
    c. Non-ventilated sections of lung result in increased dead space
    d. Alveolar PaO_2 is greater than arterial PaO_2 in normal lungs

22. Regarding the fluid compartments
    a. The plasma contains more protein than the interstitial fluid
    b. Intracellular proteins exert a positive charge at physiological pH
    c. The Donnan equilibrium influences the movement of calcium ions
    d. Transcellular fluid compartments include the CSF and GI secretions

23. Airway resistance in asthma is increased by the following
    a. Elevated bronchial smooth muscle tone as a result of increased sympathetic activity
    b. The development of turbulent airflow in the large airways
    c. Increased lung compliance secondary to hyperinflation
    d. Decreased airway calibre secondary to increased secretions

24. Facial nerve
    a. This emerges from the stylomastoid foramen
    b. It has six terminal branches that all arise distal to the parotid gland
    c. Damage to the buccal branch results in weakness of the muscles of the lower lip
    d. The cervical branch supplies platysma

25. Factors that adversely affect the healing of a wound include the following:
    a. Vitamin C deficiency
    b. Apposition of the edges
    c. Glucocorticoids
    d. Deficiency of sulphur-containing amino acids

26. **Lithium**
    a. This has a narrow therapeutic index
    b. Toxicity is exacerbated by hyponatraemia, and concurrent use of diuretics, especially thiazides, should be avoided
    c. It may be useful in the treatment of Wernicke's encephalopathy
    d. Toxic effects commonly include headache, urinary retention and rashes

27. **The following results from venous blood analysis are given for a patient in the emergency department (ED)**

Na^+	135 μmol/L
K^+	3.0 μmol/L
Urea	7.5 μmol/L
Creatinine	80 μmol/L
Cl^-	112 μmol/L
pH	7.2
$PaCO_2$	4.5 kPa (33.8 mmHg)
HCO_3^-	10.0 μmol/L

    Which of the following statements is/are likely to be true?
    a. The patient has a respiratory acidosis
    b. Diabetic ketoacidosis is the most likely cause
    c. The anion gap is 16 mmol/L
    d. The patient may have ingested acetazolamide

28. **Vasopressin**
    a. It is released directly from the brain in a circadian fashion
    b. It is released from the posterior pituitary in response to reduced plasma osmolarity
    c. Alcohol antagonises the actions of vasopressin in the kidney
    d. Vasopressin release is stimulated by angiotensin II

29. **The following are spread by the faecal–oral route**
    a. Hepatitis D
    b. Hepatitis E
    c. Hepatitis B
    d. Hepatitis A

30. **During the cardiac cycle the following statements are true**
    a. The left ventricular end-diastolic pressure is dependent on the pulmonary venous pressure
    b. The right ventricular end-diastolic pressure is dependent on the central venous pressure
    c. The end-diastolic volume will be less if there is decreased compliance of the ventricular wall
    d. If the end-diastolic volume increases, the force of contraction always decreases

31. **Cholecystokinin**
    a. This is predominantly released from the duodenum
    b. It is released in response to dietary carbohydrates
    c. It stimulates gastric parietal cells
    d. It promotes gastric emptying

32. **Regarding lipid-regulating drugs**
    a. The statins (such as simvastatin and atorvastatin) act by stimulating lipoprotein lipase activity
    b. Statins reduce plasma cholesterol by increasing the number of LDL receptors
    c. The major side effects of statins are a risk of renal failure and headache
    d. Statins can safely be given in pregnancy

33. **Paracetamol (acetaminophen)**
    a. This is principally metabolised by the liver and eliminated by the kidneys
    b. It probably has its analgesic action by an indirect action on μ receptors in the brain stem
    c. It has N-acetylbenzoquinoneimine as a toxic metabolite, which is inactivated by glutathione
    d. When taken in overdose, the drug N-acetylcysteine should be administered immediately

34. **Blood transfusions**
    a. Those who are blood group 'O positive' are considered universal donors
    b. ABO incompatibility will present with cardiovascular collapse due to haemolysis, usually after 12 hours
    c. Isolated pyrexia in the recipient of a blood transfusion may be due to white cell antibodies
    d. Jaundice may present more than 7 days after a transfusion

35. **Concerning syphilis**
    a. The incidence is decreasing in the UK
    b. The presence of a widespread rash is likely to indicate tertiary syphilis
    c. The primary chancre is usually painful
    d. The treatment regimen may depend on the patient's HIV status

36. **Which of the following may result in a defective human immune response?**
    a. Viral infections
    b. Treatment with propylthiouracil
    c. Old age
    d. Obesity

37. Loop diuretics
a. These include furosemide and bendroflumethiazide
b. They work by inhibiting NaCl reabsorption in the thick ascending loop of Henle
c. They work only in acute decompensated heart failure after a significant diuresis has been achieved
d. They may cause irreversible deafness

38. In glycolysis
a. The main compound formed is acetyl-CoA
b. Insulin will inhibit glycolysis
c. Low levels of intracellular ATP will stimulate glycolysis
d. Adrenaline (epinephrine) will stimulate glycolysis

39. Which of the following may cause chronic hepatitis?
a. Hepatitis A
b. Wilson's disease
c. Treatment with amiodarone
d. SLE

40. In head injuries
a. Tachycardia and hypotension result from rising intracranial pressure
b. Pupil dilatation occurs on the contralateral side to an intracranial haematoma
c. Autoregulation may be lost
d. Normocapnia should be aimed for in ventilated patients

41. Features of an acute myocardial infarction on an ECG that are recognised indications for thrombolysis include the following
a. ST elevation of ≥ 1 mm in V5 and V6
b. Left bundle-branch block
c. ST elevation of ≥ 2 mm in two or more contiguous chest leads
d. New right bundle-branch block

42. Chest radiograph findings in aortic dissection include the following
a. Widened mediastinum
b. Right-sided pleural effusion
c. Leftward tracheal deviation
d. Double aortic knuckle

43. Von Willebrand's disease
a. This is a family of disorders that together represent the most common inherited bleeding disorder
b. It commonly presents with epistaxis and menorrhagia
c. It may be acquired secondary to hypothyroidism
d. The bleeding time is usually abnormal

44. **The ulnar nerve**
    a. This is the terminal branch of the anterior cord of the brachial plexus
    b. It supplies all the intrinsic muscles of the hand
    c. If damaged it results in paraesthesia of the medial $2\frac{1}{2}$ digits
    d. Injury leads to wrist drop

45. **Criteria for transfer to a regional burns unit include the following**
    a. Full-thickness burns of greater than 5% of the body surface area
    b. Patients with burns and type 1 diabetes
    c. 3% partial-thickness burns over the perineum
    d. 3% partial-thickness burns in a child aged 4 years

46. **Regarding confidence intervals when analysing data from a clinical trial**
    a. A 95% confidence interval gives a range around the trial data within which we can be 95% sure that the true value lies
    b. A 95% confidence interval is calculated as 1 standard deviation either side of the trial result
    c. The wider the confidence interval the more likely that the trial result is true
    d. Confidence intervals assume the use of parametric data

47. **Giardiasis**
    a. This is a diarrhoeal disease of the colon
    b. It is an important cause of travellers' diarrhoea
    c. It is caused by an anaerobic bacterium
    d. It may cause steatorrhoea

48. **The anterior upper arm**
    a. Contains biceps, coracobrachialis and brachialis, the combined action of which flexes the arm
    b. The muscles of the anterior arm are supplied by the musculocutaneous nerve
    c. The biceps tendon lies medial to the brachial artery at the elbow
    d. The musculocutaneous nerve terminates as the lateral cutaneous nerve of the forearm

49. **Regarding scabies**
    a. Intense itching occurs at the time of infection
    b. Treatment should include all family members
    c. There is no need to change clothes/bed linen
    d. A typically infested person has thousands of mites

50. **Axillary nerve damage**
    a. This may occur in anterior dislocation of the glenohumeral joint
    b. It commonly occurs in mid-shaft humeral fractures
    c. It results in weakness of deltoid and teres minor muscles
    d. There is no sensory loss

11. Mock examination 2: Answers

1a. T
1b. F
1c. F
1d. T
The femoral sheath is a fascial tube that extends 3–4 cm inferior to the inguinal ligament. It encloses the proximal part of the femoral vessels and the femoral canal. The femoral nerve lies outside the sheath on the lateral aspect. The femoral sheath has three compartments: the lateral compartment contains the femoral artery, the intermediate compartment contains the femoral vein, and the medial compartment (femoral canal) contains connective tissue, fat, lymph vessels and sometimes a deep inguinal lymph node (Cloquet's node). The base of the femoral canal is called the femoral ring.

2a. F
2b. F
2c. T
2d. T
Eighty per cent of circulating cortisol is bound to cortisol-binding globulin, 10% to albumin, and the remainder is free and active. Cortisol secretion follows a circadian rhythm, peaking just before waking and declining as the day progresses. Stress, both emotional and physical, increases corticotrophin-releasing hormone (CRH) secretion from the hypothalamus and hence raises cortisol secretion.

3a. F
3b. F
3c. T
3d. T
The following virus and disease pairings are correct:

- Varicella-zoster – chickenpox
- EBV (Epstein–Barr virus) – glandular fever
- Parvovirus B19 – slapped-cheek syndrome or erythema infectiosum
- Paromyxovirus – measles.

4a. F
4b. F
4c. F
4d. F
The femoral artery arises from the external iliac artery. The main branch of the femoral artery is the deep artery of the thigh. The femoral artery becomes the popliteal artery as it passes through the adductor canal. It is the popliteal artery that divides into the anterior and posterior tibial arteries. The dorsalis pedis artery arises from the anterior tibial artery distal to the inferior extensor retinaculum at the ankle joint.

5a. T
5b. F
5c. T
5d. T
In AML, there is malignant proliferation of the myeloblasts in the blood and marrow. Presentation is usually with symptoms and signs of bone marrow failure and/or DIC (disseminated intravascular coagulation). Hepatospleno-megaly is common and lymphadenopathy rare. Gum infiltration is common. The myeloblasts stain positive with Sudan black and peroxidase, but negative for PAS (periodic acid–Schiff). Auer rods, when seen, are pathognomonic of AML. Treatment is with chemotherapy and bone marrow transplantation in children. Neuronal disease is unusual and IT methotrexate is rarely required. Prognosis is generally poor.

6a. F
6b. T
6c. F
6d. T
Primary hyperparathyroidism is usually caused by gland hyperplasia or a benign adenoma. It presents with features of raised calcium such as abdominal pain and polydipsia, and often radiographic evidence of bone resorption such as a pepper pot skull. In secondary hyperparathyroidism, parathyroid hormone (PTH) is chronically raised as a consequence of hypocalcaemia, as in chronic renal failure, so the calcium is usually low. In tertiary hyperparathyroidism, the function of the gland (as a result of secondary hyperparathyroidism) becomes autonomous and once again the calcium levels increase.

7a. T
7b. T
7c. F
7d. F
Avascular necrosis is seen most commonly in scaphoid fractures (particularly waist and pole fractures), lunate fractures (Kienböck's disease) and intra-capsular neck of femur fractures.

8a. T
8b. F
8c. F
8d. T
Hypochromia is the poor uptake of stain into the red cells, making them appear less dense. It is commonly seen in films of patients with iron deficiency but may also be seen in individuals with thalassaemia and patients with side-roblastic anaemia. Basophilic stippling, although commonly seen in lead poi-soning, is also associated with thalassaemia and other congenital anaemias. Blast cells are nucleated marrow cells found in the periphery; they are always abnormal. Poikilocytes are cells of varying shapes and are associated with iron deficiency, thalassaemia and myelofibrosis.

9a. F
9b. T
9c. T
9d. F
Likelihood ratios are powerful tools for assessing diagnostic accuracy of a test and are more clinically applicable than many other statistics. They are calculated using the sensitivity and specificity of a test:

Positive likelihood ratio (LR+) = sensitivity/(1 − specificity)
Negative likelihood ratio (LR−) = (1 − sensitivity)/specificity

A likelihood ratio >1 indicates that the test result is associated with disease and <1 that the test result is associated with absence of disease. However, it is not until LR+ >5 and LR− <0.2 that they become most useful. The likelihood ratios can be applied to a pre-test probability (most easily using a nomogram) to estimate the post-test probability.

10a. F
10b. T
10c. F
10d. T
Cushing's syndrome results from glucocorticoid excess, either exogenously administered (the most common cause) or endogenously produced. Cushing's disease refers to an adrenocorticotrophic hormone (ACTH)-secreting pituitary adenoma. Excess ACTH may also be secreted ectopically from a number of tumours, including small-cell lung carcinoma.

Excess glucocorticoids inhibit osteoblast activity, leading to osteoporosis.

11a. T
11b. F
11c. F
11d. T
Flecainide is a class IC antiarrhythmic agent. It acts by blocking fast Na^+ channels, slowing repolarisation and conduction, and prolonging repolarisation and action potential duration. It has a negative inotropic effect and is therefore contraindicated in patients with poor myocardial function.

12a. F
12b. F
12c. F
12d. F
The scalp has five layers, which can be remembered using the mnemonic SCALP:

- Layer 1 is the **s**kin
- Layer 2 consists of **c**onnective tissue and the arterial blood supply of the scalp
- Layer 3 is the **a**poneurosis
- Layer 4 is made of **l**oose tissue

- Layer 5 is the pericranium: a dense layer of connective tissue that forms the external periosteum of the calvaria.

The arterial blood supply is from the external carotid artery via the occipital, posterior auricular and superficial temporal arteries, and from the internal carotid artery via the supratrochlear and supraorbital arteries. Scalp lacerations bleed profusely because the arteries entering the scalp bleed from both ends, as a result of the abundant anastomoses; in addition they do not retract when lacerated because the ends are held open by the dense connective tissue. The first three layers are intimately connected and move as a unit. Layer 4 is the danger area of the scalp because pus or blood spreads easily in it. Infections in this layer can also spread into the cranial cavity through emissary veins that pass through parietal foramina in the calvaria.

13a. T
13b. F
13c. T
13d. T
Heparin initiates anticoagulation rapidly but has a short duration of action. It has two forms: unfractionated heparin and low-molecular-weight heparins, which have a longer duration of action. Although a low-molecular-weight heparin is generally preferred for routine use, heparin can be used in those at high risk of bleeding because its effect can be terminated rapidly by stopping the infusion. The use of low-molecular-weight heparin does usually require routine monitoring of the aPTT (activated partial thromboplastin time) as the dose is given depending on weight of the patient.

The main side effects of all types of heparin include thrombocytopenia (immune mediated) and hyperkalaemia (inhibition of aldosterone secretion), so heparin should be avoided in patients who are also receiving drugs that may cause hyperkalaemia. Heparin should be stopped if the platelet count is reduced by more than 50%. Rare side effects include alopecia, skin necrosis and priapism.

14a. T
14b. T
14c. F
14d. F
The pleura forms an enclosed sac, which covers the lungs. The parietal pleura lines the rib cage and the visceral pleura encases the lungs. The potential space between the parietal and visceral pleura contains a small amount of pleural fluid, which allows the two layers to glide over each other during respiration. The apex of the pleura can extend up to 2–3 cm above the level of the medial third of the clavicle. The visceral pleura is insensitive to pain because it has no nerves of general sensation, whereas the parietal pleura is extremely sensitive to pain; this also results in referred pain in the region supplied by the same segment of the spinal cord.

15a. F
15b. T
15c. F
15d. F

Transport of carbon dioxide is predominately in plasma as bicarbonate. When bound to haemoglobin, it forms carbaminohaemoglobin (carboxyhaemoglobin is carbon monoxide and haemoglobin). Deoxygenated blood has an increased CO_2-carrying capacity because reduced (deoxygenated) Hb is a better proton acceptor (Haldane effect).

16a. F
16b. T
16c. T
16d. F

The sinoatrial (SA) node's action potential is different from that of ventricular muscle, with a more positive resting potential and slower upstroke (due to the activation of slow Ca^{2+} channels; there are no fast Na^+ channels in the SA node). Adenosine blocks the AV (atrioventricular) node and is used in the treatment of supraventricular tachycardia.

17a. T
17b. F
17c. T
17d. F

Saliva undergoes secondary modification within the salivary ducts. Sympathetic stimulation leads to a 'dry mouth'. Parasympathetic stimulation is blocked by atropine. Saliva also contains R protein, which 'protects' vitamin B_{12}, lysozyme and immunoglobulins A, G and M. Control is from the medulla oblongata via parasympathetics following cranial nerves VII and IX.

18a. T
18b. F
18c. F
18d. T

The aortic arch gives rise to the brachiocephalic artery, which divides, behind the right sternoclavicular joint, into the right common carotid artery and the right subclavian artery. The aortic arch then gives off the left common carotid artery and the left subclavian artery. The veins lie anterior to the arteries in the thoracic inlet.

19a. F
19b. T
19c. T
19d. T

Campylobacter infection is a common cause of diarrhoeal illness, typically occurring after ingestion of contaminated poultry. It causes a flu-like illness, headache and diarrhoea, which may be bloody. After infection a reactive arthritis, Reiter's syndrome or Guillain–Barré syndrome may develop.

20a. T
20b. F
20c. F
20d. T
The four regions of the stomach are the cardia (the part surrounding the cardial orifice), the fundus (the dilated superior part that is related to the left dome of the diaphragm), the body (lies between the fundus and pylorus) and the pylorus (sphincter that controls discharge of the stomach contents). The arterial supply to the stomach is via the gastric arteries, which arise from the coeliac trunk and its branches. The coeliac axis gives off three main branches: the hepatic artery, splenic artery and left gastric artery. The coeliac axis supplies the oesophagus, stomach, duodenum proximal to the bile duct, liver, biliary apparatus and pancreas. The stomach receives its parasympathetic nerve supply via the vagus nerve.

21a. T
21b. F
21c. F
21d. T
In the normal lung, ventilation is maximal at the base and decreases towards the apex; similarly blood flow through the lungs is maximal in zone 3 (the base) and deceases up to zone 1 at the apex. Non-ventilated areas of lung result in a decreased $\dot{V}/\dot{Q}$ and create a functional shunt. Non-perfused areas of lung increase the $\dot{V}/\dot{Q}$, creating functional dead space.

22a. T
22b. F
22c. F
22d. T
The plasma proteins are the only components of the plasma that do not cross into the intracellular space and these proteins have a negative charge at physiological pH. The Donnan equilibrium is concerned with the movement of chloride (Cl^-) ions.

23a. F
23b. T
23c. F
23d. T
Airway resistance is a function of flow rate, airway calibre, nature of gas breathed and type of flow (laminar vs turbulent). Bronchoconstriction (caused by parasympathetic activity), together with secretions and oedema, reduces the airway diameter. Resistance is proportional to the fourth power of the radius (Poiseuille's law). Increased turbulence of airflow occurs with increasing velocity, respiratory rate and diameter of tubing. Hyperinflation moves the lungs upwards on the pressure–volume curve, decreasing compliance (lungs stiffer).

24a. T
24b. F
24c. F
24d. T
The motor root of the facial nerve supplies the muscles of facial expression. Once the facial nerve exits the stylomastoid foramen, it gives off the posterior auricular nerve. It then enters the parotid gland. Here it forms the parotid plexus, which gives rise to the five terminal branches of the facial nerve:

1. Temporal: supplies auricularis superior and auricularis anterior, the frontal belly of occipitofrontalis and the superior part of orbicularis oculi
2. Zygomatic: supplies inferior part of orbicularis oculi and other facial muscles inferior to the orbit
3. Buccal: supplies buccinator and muscles of the upper lip
4. Marginal mandibular: supplies risorius and muscles of the lower lip and chin
5. Cervical: supplies the platysma.

25a. T
25b. F
25c. T
25d. T
Wound healing will be significantly slowed in the presence of infection and poor blood supply (diabetes). Apposition of wound edges will improve the healing.

Glucocorticoids prevent healing by inhibiting the formation of new blood vessels.

Sulphur-containing amino acids and vitamin C are both needed for the production of collagen.

26a. T
26b. T
26c. F
26d. F
The therapeutic and toxic doses of lithium are similar and patients regularly need to have their serum lithium levels checked. Many drugs can increase the likelihood of toxicity and diuretics, due to their tendency to cause hyponatraemia, and should be avoided if possible in patients on lithium. Common symptoms of toxicity include tremor, ataxia, dysarthria, nystagmus and convulsions.

27a. F
27b. F
27c. T
27d. T
Routine serum analysis measures more cations (Na^+ and K^+) than anions (Cl^- and HCO_3^-). The difference is referred to as the anion gap and is usually in the range of 10–16 mmol/L, reflecting the presence of unmeasured anions. Most states of acidosis will have a raised anion gap (lactic acidosis, renal failure,

ketosis, alcohol, diabetes, salicylate poisoning). A normal anion gap may be present in renal tubular acidosis, diarrhoea, acetazolamide poisoning, Addison's disease and ammonium chloride ingestion.

28a. T
28b. F
28c. T
28d. T

Vasopressin is derived from a pre-prohormone precursor that is synthesised in the hypothalamus and stored in vesicles at the posterior pituitary. Vasopressin is secreted from the posterior pituitary gland in response to reductions in plasma volume, and increases in the plasma osmolality and cholecystokinin secreted by the small intestine. Secretion in response to reduced plasma volume is activated by pressure receptors in the veins, atria and carotids. Secretion in response to increases in plasma osmotic pressure is mediated by osmoreceptors in the hypothalamus.

Secretion in response to increases in plasma cholecystokinin is mediated by an unknown pathway.

The neurons that make vasopressin, in the hypothalamic supraoptic nuclei (SONs) and paraventricular nuclei (PVNs), are themselves osmoreceptors, but they also receive synaptic input from other osmoreceptors located in regions adjacent to the anterior wall of the third ventricle.

Many factors influence the secretion of vasopressin:

- Ethanol (alcohol) acts as an antagonist for vasopressin in the collecting ducts of the kidneys, which prevents aquaporins from binding to the collecting ducts, and prevents water reabsorption.
- Angiotensin II may stimulate the secretion of vasopressin.

Vasopressin increases the permeability to water of the distal convoluted tubules and collecting tubules in the nephrons of kidneys, thus allowing water reabsorption and excretion of a smaller volume of concentrated urine. Vasopressin increases peripheral vascular resistance and thus increases arterial blood pressure.

Vasopressin released within the brain has many actions:

- It has been implicated in memory formation, including delayed reflexes, image, and short- and long-term memory, although the mechanism remains unknown and these findings are controversial. However, the synthetic vasopressin analogue desmopressin has come to attention as a likely nootropic.
- Vasopressin is released into the brain in a circadian rhythm by neurons of the suprachiasmatic nucleus of the hypothalamus.
- Vasopressin released from centrally projecting hypothalamic neurons is involved in aggression, blood pressure regulation and temperature regulation.

29a. F
29b. T
29c. F
29d. T
Hepatitis B, C and D are spread parenterally. Hepatitis A and E are spread by the faecal–oral route.

30a. T
30b. T
30c. F
30d. F
The force of contraction of the ventricles is related to the degree of stretch of the cardiac muscle. This is known as the Frank–Starling relationship. As the end-diastolic volume increases, the force of contraction also increases. The end-diastolic volume will depend on the compliance of the ventricular wall (the more compliant the wall, the more filling it will allow) and the end-diastolic pressure.

31a. F
31b. T
31c. F
31d. F
Excreted from jejunal mucosa in response to acid/protein loading, chole-cystokinin is a potent inhibitor of gastric emptying and secretion. It acts to contract the gallbladder and causes pancreatic secretion of enzymes. Together with gastrin, it stimulates glucagon secretion.

32a. F
32b. T
32c. F
32d. F
The statins are HMG (hydroxymethylglutaryl)-CoA reductase inhibitors and block the synthesis of cholesterol in the liver. This reduction in cholesterol leads to an increase in the number of LDL (low-density lipoprotein) receptors, which reduces the plasma cholesterol further. The most common side effects from statins are myalgia, myopathy and myositis. As cholesterol is vital for fetal development, statins should not be given during pregnancy.

33a. T
33b. F
33c. T
33d. F
Paracetamol is a highly effective analgesic that probably has its effects by inhibiting prostaglandin synthetase. It may also have an effect on prostaglandin E_2 synthesis in the hypothalamus; hence its action as an antipyretic. Parace-tamol is metabolised by conjugation reactions in the liver and ultimately excreted by the kidneys. After high doses these conjugation enzymes may become saturated, and it is then metabolised to the toxic metabolite N-acetylbenzoquinoneimine, which is inactivated by glutathione. In overdose

these glutathione stores are quickly used up and the toxic metabolite causes hepatocellular necrosis. Glutathione itself cannot be administered as an antidote because it is unable to enter cells, so a precursor, N-acetylcysteine (NAC), is given. As there is a chance of anaphylaxis with NAC, a serum paracetamol level is measured at 4 hours after ingestion and checked against a nomogram. If the paracetamol level is above the treatment line, NAC is then given. If the patient presents over 8 hours after ingestion of more than 150 mg/ kg or 12 g paracetamol, NAC may be given without waiting for a paracetamol level.

34a. F
34b. F
34c. T
34d. T
Using the ABO and rhesus blood groups, those with type 'O negative' are considered universal donors because they contain no cell membrane surface antigens for a recipient to react to. Conversely those with blood type AB positive are considered universal recipients because their blood contains no antibodies to the A, B or rhesus antigens.

Severe ABO mismatch will result in immediate shock, fever and haemolysis, which is potentially fatal. Isolated pyrexias are often due to white cell antibody reactions and usually occur in the first 1–2 hours. Mismatch to minor red cell antibodies can present late (often 7–10 days) and symptoms include anaemia, jaundice and fever.

35a. F
35b. F
35c. F
35d. T
Syphilis is caused by infection with the spirochaete *Treponema pallidum*. There are four stages:

1. Painless primary chancre usually on the mouth or genitals
2. Rash and lymphadenopathy (positive serology)
3. Organ disruption (negative serology)
4. General paralysis.

Treatment needs to be more aggressive in those who are HIV positive and neurosyphilis is far more common in these individuals.

36a. T
36b. T
36c. T
36d. F
The immune system may be impaired by many agents. Infection (bacterial, viral and fungal) may cause leukopenia. Many drugs affect the immune system, e.g. chemotherapy, antibiotics, steroids, and antifungal and antithyroid drugs. The extremes of age adversely affect the function of the immune system, as does malnutrition.

37a. F
37b. T
37c. F
37d. T
Loop diuretics such as furosemide and bumetanide act on the luminal membrane of the thick ascending loop of Henle, inhibiting the co-transport of $Na^+/K^+/2Cl^-$, and resulting in significant renal salt and water excretion. The first therapeutic effects seen in acute decompensated heart failure are via neurohumerally mediated venodilatation, and they occur much faster than the diuretic effect. They may cause irreversible deafness in large concentrations via changes in the electrolyte composition of the endolymph.

38a. F
38b. F
38c. T
38d. F
Glycolysis is the splitting of glucose in the cytosol of all cells in the body. It is the archetypal universal metabolic pathway. It occurs, with variations, in almost all organisms, both aerobic and anaerobic. Aerobic metabolism of one molecule of glucose will result in two molecules of ATP, two molecules of pyruvate and two molecules of NADH (which in turn can each produce three molecules of ATP when they are further reduced to $NADH_2$). The pyruvate generated is then available for the tricarboxylic or citric acid cycle, which occurs in the mitochondria. Anaerobic glycolysis increases the production of lactate with a reduced yield of ATP. Intracellular regulators include amino acids, the citric acid cycle intermediate citrate, and the acyl intermediates acetyl-CoA and fatty acids. All will stimulate gluconeogenesis and inhibit glycolysis. In addition, the energy charge of cells controls glycolysis and gluconeogenesis, with low energy levels (AMP, ADP) stimulating glycolysis and high energy levels (ATP) inhibiting glycolysis and activating gluconeogenesis.

Hormones are extracellular regulators that also affect glycolysis and gluconeogenesis. They coordinate metabolic activity among different organs. Insulin stimulates glycolysis to lower blood glucose levels after a meal, which signals that energy is available to all organs, whereas glucagon and adrenaline (epinephrine) stimulate gluconeogenesis (and lipolysis in fatty tissue by hepatic lipase) to provide energy to the muscle and brain during stress. Gluconeogenesis is essentially the opposite of glycolysis except that it occurs mainly in liver cells. The most common substrate is lactate (via pyruvate through the Cori [glucose–lactate] cycle using lactate dehydrogenase), but amino acids can also be converted to glucose, as can uneven-chain fatty acids.

39a. F
39b. T
39c. T
39d. F
Hepatitis A is usually a short-lived infection that may rarely cause severe hepatitis but not chronic hepatitis, as the virus is usually cleared. Wilson's disease results in copper deposition in organs and the liver is commonly affected. Amiodarone in chronic use may result in cirrhosis and chronic

hepatitis, although this is rare. SLE (systemic lupus erythematosus) does not affect the liver.

40a. F
40b. F
40c. T
40d. T
In head injuries, autoregulation maintaining the cerebral perfusion pressure over a range of blood pressures is lost. An expanding temporal lobe haematoma causes uncal transtentorial herniation, compressing the oculomotor nerve, and causing ipsilateral pupil dilatation. With rises in intracranial pressure, the Cushing reflex results in increasing blood pressure and bradycardia. In ventilated patients normocapnia should be the goal, so as to avoid cerebral artery vasoconstriction.

41a. F
41b. T
41c. T
41d. F
The ECG changes considered to be an indication for thrombolysis are:

- ST elevation of ≥ 1 mm in two limb leads
- ST elevation of ≥ 2 mm in two or more contiguous chest leads (V1, V2, V3, V4, V5, V6)
- Left bundle-branch block (does not have to be new) in the presence of a history typical of acute myocardial infarction.

42a. T
42b. F
42c. F
42d. T
The only definitive test for aortic dissection is computed tomography (CT) and this should be performed in any patient in whom the diagnosis is being considered. There may be several signs present on a plain chest radiograph that increase the likelihood of aortic dissection: widened mediastinum, left-sided pleural effusion, right-sided tracheal deviation, and a double aortic knuckle. It should be remembered that 12% of patients with aortic dissection will have a normal chest radiograph (and about 30% will have a normal ECG), so these tests alone are insufficient to rule out the diagnosis – they are poorly sensitive.

43a. T
43b. T
43c. T
43d. T
von Willebrand's disease (vWD) has up to 22 subtypes but together they represent the most common inherited bleeding disorder. In the most common autosomal dominant form (chromosome 12), there is a deficiency of von Willebrand's factor (vWF), which acts as a carrier protein for factor VIII. vWF is also required for normal platelet function.

In those patients with vWD, there will be an elevated aPTT and bleeding time. It usually presents with increased or easy bruising, recurrent epistaxis, menorrhagia and postoperative bleeding (particularly after tonsillectomy or dental extractions). Many children with vWD are asymptomatic and diagnosed as a result of a positive family history. Rare acquired forms of the disease can be due to Wilms' tumour, congenital heart disease, SLE, angiodysplasia or hypothyroidism.

44a. F
44b. F
44c. F
44d. F
The ulnar nerve originates from the medial cord of the brachial plexus. It supplies all the intrinsic muscles of the hand except the lateral two lumbricals and the muscles of the thenar eminence. It transmits sensation from the ulnar $1\frac{1}{2}$ fingers. Wrist drop occurs with a radial nerve palsy whereas an injury to the ulnar nerve results in claw hand.

45a. T
45b. T
45c. T
45d. F
Several organisations have produced guidance (including the American Burn Association and the UK National Burn Care Review) on which patients should be transferred to a regional burns centre. This may vary between burn centres, but any question in the MCEM should be unambiguous. The most up-to-date guidance is from the American Burn Association (and also used in ATLS – Advanced Trauma Life Support) and includes:

- Partial-thickness and full-thickness burns on >10% of the body surface area (BSA) in patients <10 years or >50 years of age
- Partial-thickness and full-thickness burns on >20% of the BSA in other age groups
- Partial-thickness and full-thickness burns involving the face, eyes, ears, hands, feet, genitalia and perineum, as well as those that involve skin overlying major joints
- Full-thickness burns on >5% of the BSA in any age group
- Significant electrical burns, including lightning injury
- Significant chemical burns
- Inhalational injury
- Burn injury in patients with pre-existing illness that could complicate treatment, prolong recovery or affect mortality.

46a. T
46b. F
46c. F
46d. T
A trial can use a sample only to try to reflect the whole population being studied. Confidence intervals help us tell how much certainty there is around the result obtained in a trial. The narrower the confidence interval the

more certain we can be that the trial result is precise. Confidence intervals are usually expressed as 95% or approximately 2 standard deviations either side of the trial result. They are useful only in parametric (normally distributed) data.

47a. F
47b. T
47c. F
47d. T
Giardiasis, a disease of the small bowel, is a result of infection by a flagellate protozoan *Giardia lamblia*. It damages the small bowel villi, causing malabsorption and diarrhoea. It does cause travellers' diarrhoea but person-to-person spread is also common in communal institutions.

48a. T
48b. T
48c. F
48d. T
As well as flexing the arm, biceps also supinates the forearm. Coracobrachialis also adducts the arm. The musculocutaneous nerve arises from the lateral cord of the brachial plexus and supplies the muscles of the anterior upper arm before terminating as the lateral cutaneous nerve of the forearm, which transmits sensation from the lateral aspect of the forearm. The biceps tendon lies lateral to the brachial artery at the elbow.

49a. F
49b. T
49c. F
49d. F
Scabies is a dermatophilic infestation by the mite *Sarcoptes scabiei*. A papular rash and itching occur about 6 weeks from infection due to the development of sensitivity to the mite faeces and saliva. Typically infestations are with 10–15 live female mites. Norwegian or crusted scabies involves infection with thousands/millions of mites and is seen in the immunocompromised host. Treatment involves topical application of an ascaricide to the entire household. All clothing and bed linen should be cleaned.

50a. T
50b. F
50c. T
50d. F
The axillary nerve is easily damaged in anterior dislocations of the glenohumeral joint. In mid-shaft humeral fractures, the radial nerve is more commonly injured than the axillary nerve. The axillary nerve supplies a patch of skin over the inferior part of the deltoid muscle.

12. Mock examination 3: Questions

1. Hypokalaemia
   a. This may result from the action of insulin
   b. It is caused by excess aldosterone
   c. It is associated with β-blocker use
   d. It stimulates renin release

2. The median nerve
   a. This supplies all the flexor muscles of the forearm
   b. It is compressed in cubital tunnel syndrome
   c. It innervates the muscles of the thenar eminence
   d. It transmits sensation from the palm and the anterior surface
      and distal third of the posterior surface of the radial $3\frac{1}{2}$ fingers

3. Within the cell
   a. Lysosomes manufacture enzymes that enable the production of
      hydrogen ions
   b. The endoplasmic reticulum is formed of multiple areas of Golgi
      apparatus and is the site for processing newly made proteins
   c. The nucleus contains liquid known as karyolymph, a nucleolus
      and chromatin (which contains the cell's DNA)
   d. Half of the content of the cell is made up of a viscous, lipid-rich
      fluid called cytosol

4. The following conditions may result in a raised alkaline
   phosphatase (ALP)
   a. Paget's disease
   b. Osteosarcoma
   c. Hyperparathyroidism
   d. Pregnancy

5. The coronary arteries
   a. The right coronary artery (RCA) arises from the right coronary
      sinus on the pulmonary artery
   b. The two main branches of the RCA are the right marginal
      branch and the posterior descending artery
   c. The RCA supplies the sinoatrial node in 30% of the population
   d. The two main branches of the left coronary artery (LCA) are
      the circumflex and the left anterior descending artery

6. **In Hodgkin's lymphoma**
   a. A raised ESR would indicate a worse prognosis
   b. Stage 2 disease (Ann Arbor classification) will affect lymph nodes above and below the diaphragm
   c. Patients with nodular sclerosing cell type have a worse prognosis
   d. Patients may present with hepatosplenomegaly

7. **Cerebral hemispheres**
   a. The motor cortex lies in the posterior part of the pre-central gyrus
   b. The sensory cortex lies in the post-central gyrus
   c. Lesions in Wernicke's area result in expressive dysphasia
   d. The visual cortex lies on the occipital pole

8. **Pertussis (whooping cough)**
   a. This is a contagious viral illness
   b. It is a notifiable disease
   c. It is rare in adolescents and adults
   d. It causes apnoea in young babies

9. **Calcium absorption is increased by the following**
   a. Calcium deficiency
   b. Consumption of foods high in oxalate
   c. Consumption of a high protein diet
   d. 1,25-Dihydroxycholecalciferol

10. **Surfactant**
    a. This contains mucopolypeptides
    b. It prevents oedema formation within alveoli
    c. It acts to increase lung compliance
    d. It reduces surface tension

11. **Femoral nerve**
    a. This arises from L2–4
    b. It enters the thigh on the medial side of the femoral artery
    c. It supplies the posterior compartment of the thigh
    d. It has no sensory branches

12. **When a wound heals by secondary intention**
    a. The wound edges are usually opposed
    b. The process involves contraction of the wound that is caused by the collagen fibres
    c. The scar is generally worse than with primary intention
    d. Granulation tissue forms from the edges and base of the wound

13. The following are physiological causes of oedema
a. Increased capillary pressure
b. Decreased venous pressure
c. Decreased hydrostatic pressure
d. Decreased lymph drainage

14. Conduction of electrical impulses throughout the heart
a. The conduction commences at the sinoatrial node
b. The electrical impulses spread through the atria via the Purkinje fibres
c. They are prevented from reaching the ventricles by the annulus femoralis
d. The process is modulated by the autonomic nervous system

15. Sensory nerve supply of the face
a. The sensory information from the face is transmitted via the trigeminal nerve
b. The maxillary division of the trigeminal nerve has four cutaneous branches
c. The skin over the nose is supplied solely by the maxillary division of the trigeminal nerve
d. Lesions on the tip of the nose in shingles suggest ocular involvement

16. Glucagon
a. This acts as a positive inotrope
b. It is released from β cells in the pancreas
c. It increases the production of free fatty acids
d. It increases glycogen synthesis

17. The enteric nervous system
a. The submucous plexus innervates the smooth muscle layers of the gut
b. The myenteric plexus is responsible for control of secretions
c. Peristalsis requires input from the autonomic nervous system
d. Vagal stimulation results in gastrin secretion

18. Accelerated (malignant) or very severe hypertension
a. This requires immediate intravenous therapy
b. A β blocker such as atenolol would be an appropriate first agent
c. It may cause blindness if blood pressure is reduced too quickly
d. It is associated with a previous history of myocardial infarction

19. The following are RNA viruses
a. *Chlamydia*
b. CMV
c. Measles
d. Rubella

20. **Polycythaemia**
    a. Polycythaemia vera is a malignant marrow stem cell disorder
    b. Renal carcinoma may be the sole cause
    c. It may be associated with smoking
    d. The condition may present with epistaxis or bleeding gums

21. **Lidocaine**
    a. This has a duration of action of approximately 2 hours after intravenous injection
    b. It is not useful orally as it is largely inactivated by first-pass hepatic metabolism
    c. It is the drug of choice to treat ventricular arrhythmias after myocardial infarction
    d. It works by blocking inactivated K^+ channels

22. **Lung compliance**
    a. This is defined as the change in flow rate per unit change in pressure
    b. It is increased in emphysema
    c. It depends on lung volume
    d. It is increased in early pulmonary oedema

23. **The large intestine**
    a. The psoas muscle is closely related to the caecum
    b. It is supplied by the inferior mesenteric artery from the distal third of the transverse colon
    c. It receives its sympathetic supply from T10–L2
    d. McBurney's point is one-third of the way along the oblique line joining the umbilicus and the right anteroinferior iliac spine

24. **β-Adrenergic receptors**
    a. These may be excitatory or inhibitory
    b. They are of two main types:

       1. Type 1, which are located in the heart and airways
       2. Type 2, which are located in the peripheral vasculature

    c. When stimulated they cause a release of intracellular cyclic AMP via activation of adenylyl cyclase
    d. They may be blocked by drugs that are used in the treatment of asthma

25. **Compartments of the hand**
    a. There are five compartments in the hand
    b. There are two potential spaces in the hand
    c. The compartments prevent the spread of infection from the hand to the forearm
    d. The fibrous lateral septum divides the central and thenar compartment and runs from the lateral border of the palmar aponeurosis to the second metacarpal

26. **Adrenal gland**
    a. Adrenaline (epinephrine) is secreted from the adrenal medulla
    b. The adrenal cortex produces corticosteroids from cholesterol
    c. Aldosterone is produced from the innermost layer of the adrenal cortex
    d. Cortisol is produced from the outermost layer of the adrenal gland

27. **Regarding the cavernous sinus**
    a. Cranial nerves III (oculomotor), IV (trochlear) and VI (abducens) pass through the cavernous sinus
    b. The internal carotid artery passes through the sinus
    c. The sinus receives venous drainage from the face
    d. Thrombophlebitis can result in meningitis

28. **The following antibiotics are used in the treatment of community-acquired pneumonia**
    a. Cefotaxime
    b. Ciprofloxacin
    c. Amoxicillin
    d. Erythromycin

29. **In paroxysmal nocturnal haemoglobinuria (PNH)**
    a. A urine specimen taken at 07:00 will be light in colour
    b. Red cells are extremely sensitive to immunoglobulin, resulting in intravascular haemolysis and haemoglobinuria
    c. PNH may present with Budd–Chiari syndrome
    d. Stem cell transplantation may be curative

30. **Insulin**
    a. It increases amino acid uptake in skeletal muscle
    b. It increases protein catabolism
    c. It reduces hunger
    d. It decreases lipolysis

31. **The urinary tract**
    a. The right kidney usually lies slightly inferior to the left kidney
    b. Renal pathology may result in hip joint pain
    c. Fractures of the bony pelvis, especially those resulting from separation of the pubic symphysis and puboprostatic ligaments, usually rupture the intermediate part of the urethra
    d. Straddle injuries most commonly rupture the spongy urethra

32. *Helicobacter pylori*
    a. Infection is nearly always symptomatic
    b. *H. pylori* secretes urease
    c. It attaches to mucus via a flagellum
    d. It is associated with an increased risk of stomach cancer

33. **When looking at a differential white cell count**
    a. The neutrophil count may be increased as a result of trauma
    b. The neutrophil count may be decreased in vitamin B_{12} deficiency
    c. Fungal infections can result in a raised lymphocyte count
    d. A raised eosinophil count is pathognomonic of anaphylaxis

34. **The following are the results of a trial of the diagnostic test 'Procalysis' in the diagnosis of ischaemic heart disease**

	Ischaemic heart disease	
Procalysis	Present	Absent
Positive	200	50
Negative	300	150

    a. There were 50 true positives
    b. The number of false negatives is fewer than the number of false positives
    c. The number of people with the disease in this trial was 250
    d. The specificity of Procalysis to detect ischaemic heart disease is 50% (150/300)

35. **The following drugs may cause bradycardia**
    a. Amitriptyline
    b. Sotalol
    c. Clonidine
    d. Digoxin

36. **Diabetes insipidus**
    a. This may occur after a head injury
    b. Most patients will have polyuria and polydipsia
    c. The plasma osmolarity will be low
    d. It may be secondary to lithium therapy

37. **Multiple myeloma**
    a. This is a T-cell malignancy
    b. Hypercalcaemia is common
    c. The ESR is moderately raised
    d. Lytic lesions are commonly seen on radiograph

38. **In the treatment of diabetes mellitus**
    a. Metformin may cause a normal anion gap acidosis
    b. Metformin rarely causes hypoglycaemia
    c. Sulphonylureas require some functioning β cells to be effective
    d. Metformin requires some functioning β cells to be effective

39. Tetanus
a. The causative wound/injury is always obvious
b. Intravenous drug users are a high-risk group
c. A surgical airway is often needed if the patient suffers a cardiac arrest
d. Once affected, a patient will have life-long immunity

40. Collagen
a. This is synthesised by fibroclasts
b. It provides strength to tendons
c. Osteogenesis imperfecta results from defective type IV collagen
d. It requires vitamin C for its synthesis

41. Regarding the nerve supply to the lower limb
a. Damage to the femoral nerve results in anaesthesia to the posterior thigh
b. Compression of the sciatic nerve causes weakness of knee flexion
c. The tibial nerve is commonly injured in fractures of proximal fibula
d. Superficial peroneal nerve injury results in sensory loss to the first toe web space

42. Sodium bicarbonate
a. 50 mL of 8.4% solution contains 50 mmol bicarbonate
b. This can be given combined with calcium chloride in the treatment of hyperkalaemia
c. It may exacerbate intracellular acidosis
d. It may be useful in the treatment of β-blocker overdose

43. Aortic dissection
a. This is associated with Marfan's syndrome
b. It is associated with heroin use
c. It may present with a hemiplegia and mimic a stroke
d. Most patients are hypertensive at presentation

44. The concomitant use of which of these medications will increase bleeding risk in patients on warfarin?
a. Metronidazole
b. Paracetamol
c. Fluoxetine
d. Aspirin

45. In a normal distribution
a. The mean is the same as the mode
b. The mean is higher than the median
c. 95% of observations lie within 1 standard deviation of the mean
d. The Mann–Whitney test is suitable for analysis

46. **Knee joint**
    a. The menisci are attached to the collateral ligaments
    b. The popliteus muscle locks the knee joint
    c. The anterior cruciate ligament runs from the anterior aspect of the tibial plateau to the medial aspect of the medial femoral condyle
    d. The knee has six bursae, two of which communicate with the joint capsule

47. **The following results are given for a patient in the emergency department (ED)**

pH	7.28
PaO_2	9.5 kPa (71 mmHg)
$PaCO_2$	7.5 kPa (56 mmHg)
HCO_3^-	36.0 mmol/L
BE	−3.8
Lactate	2.4 mmol/L

    Which of the following statements is/are likely to be true?
    a. The patient has a metabolic acidosis
    b. The patient may have a reduced GCS
    c. There is no evidence of acid–base compensation
    d. The patient should be given high-flow oxygen

48. **Immune system**
    a. Macrophages are circulating polymorphonuclear cells
    b. Complement acts as an opsonin
    c. Dendritic cells and natural killer cells form part of the innate immune system
    d. B cells are the predominant lymphocytes

49. *Staphylococcus aureus*
    a. This is a Gram-positive coccus
    b. Food poisoning occurs approximately 48 hours after its ingestion
    c. It is coagulase negative
    d. It colonises the noses of up to 25% of healthy individuals

50. **Catecholamines**
    a. Noradrenaline (norepinephrine) causes vasoconstriction via β_1-receptors
    b. Adrenaline (epinephrine) dilates blood vessels in skeletal muscle
    c. β_2-Receptor stimulation increases heart rate and contractility
    d. Noradrenaline is the principal hormone secreted from the adrenal medulla

12. Mock examination 3: Answers

1a. T
1b. T
1c. F
1d. T
Hypokalaemia results from either depletion/loss of potassium, secondary to intracellular shifts of potassium. Potassium moves into cells under the influence of insulin and β_2-adrenergic agonists such as adrenaline (epinephrine) and salbutamol.

Renal potassium loss occurs in renal tubular acidosis, diabetic ketoacidosis (DKA) and excess aldosterone secretion, and by the effect of loop and thiazide diuretics.

Lowered potassium levels result in secretion of renin and hence raised angiotensin levels.

2a. F
2b. F
2c. T
2d. T
The median nerve supplies all the flexors of the forearm except flexor carpi ulnaris and the ulnar half of flexor digitorum profundus. The median nerve can be compressed in the carpal tunnel; the ulnar nerve would be compressed in the cubital tunnel. (The cubital tunnel is formed by the tendon connecting the humeral and ulnar heads of flexor carpi ulnaris.) In the hand the median nerve supplies the muscle of the thenar eminence (abductor pollicis brevis, flexor pollicis brevis and opponens pollicis) and the two radial lumbricals. The palmar branch of the median nerve, which transmits sensation from the central palm, arises proximal to the carpal tunnel and passes superficial to the flexor retinaculum. This branch can be damaged in superficial laceration of the wrist but is spared in carpal tunnel syndrome.

3a. F
3b. F
3c. T
3d. F
Each area of the cell performs a distinct function. The lysosomes are vesicles arising from the endoplasmic reticulum that are involved with the intracellular digestion of macromolecules. The Golgi apparatus is distinct from the endoplasmic reticulum and processes its products. Cytosol is a protein-rich fluid that surrounds and bathes all other components of the cell.

4a. T
4b. T
4c. T
4d. T
ALP is raised in bone disease, hyperparathyroidism, growing children and biliary hepatic disorders.

5a. F
5b. T
5c. F
5d. T
The RCA arises from the right coronary sinus on the aorta. In 60% of the population the RCA supplies the sinoatrial (SA) node with the LCA supplying the other 40%. The RCA descends in the coronary grove and gives off the right marginal branch, which supplies the right heart border. The RCA then turns left and continues in the coronary groove to the posterior aspect of the heart. On the posterior aspect of the heart, the RCA supplies the atrioventricular (AV) node in 80% of the population and then terminates as the posterior descending artery. The posterior descending artery runs down the posterior interventricular groove towards the apex of the heart. Around the apex the RCA anastomoses with branches of the LCA. The LCA arises from the left aortic sinus of the aorta. It passes alongside the pulmonary trunk. At the left heart border the LCA divides into two branches: the circumflex artery and the left anterior descending artery (LAD). The LAD runs along the anterior interventricular groove, passes round the inferior border of the heart, and anastomoses with the RCA branches.

6a. T
6b. F
6c. F
6d. T
Hodgkin's lymphoma is a malignancy of Reed–Sternberg lymphocytes. It affects young adults and elderly people, and is more common in men. It usually presents with painless lymphadenopathy, the neck being the most common site. It may present with constitutional symptoms such as weight loss, night sweats and fever, which would worsen the prognosis for any classification group, as would a raised ESR (erythrocyte sedimentation rate) and the presence of anaemia. Hypercalcaemia is common and in late disease hepatosplenomegaly may be present. Diagnosis is usually based on lymph node biopsy, and Ann Arbor staging depends on where the disease is identified:

Stage I: confined to a single region
Stage II: confined to two regions on the same side as the diaphragm
Stage III: disease both sides of the diaphragm
Stage IV: extra-lymph node disease.

The cell type also has a prognostic significance. Nodular sclerosing, mixed cellularity and lymphocyte-predominant types also have relatively good prognoses but lymphocyte-depleted disease has a poor prognosis.

7a. T
7b. T
7c. F
7d. T

The gyri are the folds in the cerebral hemispheres and the grooves are called sulci. The motor cortex lies just anterior to the central sulcus and the sensory cortex lies just posterior to the central sulcus. The auditory cortex lies on the superior border of the superior temporal gyrus. Broca's area lies in the posterior part of the inferior frontal gyrus and, if damaged, results in expressive dysphasia. Wernicke's area is in the posterior part of the superior temporal gyrus and a lesion would result in receptive dysphasia. Broca's and Wernicke's areas are found unilaterally in the brain in the dominant hemisphere, which is usually the left hemisphere. They are both supplied by the middle cerebral artery.

8a. F
8b. T
8c. F
8d. T

Pertussis is caused by the Gram-negative bacillus *Bordetella pertussis*. Infection in infants may cause apnoeic episodes and younger patients may also lack the 'whoop'.

Older patients commonly lack immunity (it decreases with time post-immunisation), and one should always consider pertussis in adults with prolonged cough and post-tussive vomiting. It is diagnosed by culture of nasopharyngeal swabs.

9a. T
9b. F
9c. T
9d. T

Absorption of calcium occurs in the duodenum/proximal jejunum. Absorption is controlled by vitamin D (1,25-dihydroxycholecalciferol), which increases calcium-binding proteins in the gut. Calcium combines with oxalate to form insoluble salts, decreasing absorption.

10a. F
10b. T
10c. T
10d. T

Surfactant, a phospholipid–protein complex, reduces surface tension to prevent alveolar collapse and oedema formation. In conditions associated with a lack of surfactant, e.g. ARDS (acute respiratory distress syndrome), the lungs are very 'stiff' (decreased compliance).

11a. T
11b. F
11c. F
11d. F
The femoral nerve lies on the lateral aspect of the femoral artery. It supplies the anterior compartment of the upper leg (hip flexors and knee extensors). The saphenous nerve is the terminal branch of the femoral nerve, and it transmits sensation from the skin on the anteromedial aspect of the thigh, knee and leg.

12a. F
12b. F
12c. T
12d. T
Wounds that heal by secondary intention have unopposed edges. Wound contraction occurs to help reduce the size of the wound and this is a function of fibroblasts. Granulation tissue forms in the wound that contains blood vessels, macrophages and fibroblasts. Maturation of the wound may take several months and the scar is often unorganised and large.

13a. T
13b. F
13c. F
13d. T
Fluid will accumulate in the interstitial space (oedema), portal venous system (ascites) and pulmonary interstitium (pulmonary oedema) if the volume of filtered blood is higher than that returned into the circulation. Increased capillary pressure will cause an increase in filtration. This effect is magnified when the capillary permeability to proteins also increases in anaphylaxis and sepsis. An increase in venous pressure or hydrostatic pressure will push fluid out of capillaries, causing oedema, e.g. in patients with deep vein thrombosis.

14a. T
14b. F
14c. F
14d. T
The heart beat is initiated by spontaneous depolarisation of the SA node, which is located in the right atrium. The electrical impulse spreads throughout the atria via gap junctions and desmosomes and is prevented from entering the ventricles by the annulus fibrosis (the annulus femoralis is a synonym for the femoral ring).

15a. T
15b. F
15c. F
15d. T
Sensory information from the face is transmitted via the three divisions of the trigeminal nerve: ophthalmic, maxillary and mandibular.

The ophthalmic division has five cutaneous branches:

1. The external nasal nerve supplies the skin on the dorsum of nose including tip of nose.
2. The infratrochlear nerve supplies the skin and conjunctiva of the upper eyelid.
3. The supratrochlear nerve supplies the skin in the middle of the forehead up to the hairline.
4. The supraorbital nerve supplies the skin of forehead and scalp, as far as the vertex of the skull, the mucous membranes of the frontal sinus, and conjunctiva of the upper eyelid.
5. The lacrimal nerve supplies the lacrimal gland and small area of skin plus conjunctiva of the lateral part of the upper eyelid.

The maxillary division has three cutaneous branches:

1. The infraorbital nerve supplies the skin of the upper cheek, the mucosa of the maxillary sinus, and the skin and conjunctiva of the inferior eyelid. It also supplies the incisor, canine and premolar teeth and adjacent upper gingiva, part of the nose, and the mucosa of the upper lip. The infraorbital nerve runs in the floor of the orbit and emerges at the infraorbital foramen; it is therefore easily damaged in blow-out fractures of the orbital floor.
2. The zygomaticotemporal nerve supplies a small area of skin over the anterior part of the temple.
3. The zygomaticofacial nerve supplies skin over the zygomatic prominence.

The mandibular division has three cutaneous branches:

1. The auriculotemporal nerve supplies the auricle, external acoustic meatus, external surface of the tympanic membrane and the skin superior to the auricle.
2. The buccal nerve supplies a thumb-size area of the skin over the cheek and supplies the mucous membrane lining the cheek and the posterior part of the buccal surface of the gingival.
3. The mental nerve supplies the skin of the chin, and the skin and mucous membrane of the lower lip and the interior labial gingiva.

Shingles (herpes zoster) is caused by herpes virus. The virus lies dormant in nerve ganglia, i.e. the trigeminal ganglia, and can be reactivated. Shingles lesions on the tip of the nose suggest involvement of the ophthalmic division of the trigeminal nerve due to the sensory distribution.

16a. T
16b. F
16c. T
16d. F
Glucagon is produced from cells in the pancreas in response to hypoglycaemia, cholecystokinin, gastrin, cortisol and sympathetic stimulation. It acts on the liver to break down glycogen and lipids, and increases gluconeogenesis from amino acids.

Large, exogenous doses of glucagon are positively inotropic by increasing myocardial cAMP.

17a. F
17b. F
17c. F
17d. T
The submucous plexus innervates the gut glandular epithelium, endocrine glands and blood vessels. The myenteric plexus controls the long and circular smooth muscle of the gut. Peristalsis, although controlled by the autonomic nervous system, occurs independently of extrinsic innervation. Parasympathetic stimulation, via the vagus, increases gastrin secretion.

18a. F
18b. T
18c. T
18d. F
Malignant hypertension (severe hypertension associated with evidence of acute and progressive damage to end organs) requires urgent treatment but is not an indication for intravenous therapy. Oral therapy, such as a β blocker or long-acting calcium channel blocker, is usually first-line. Very rarely intravenous therapy, usually with sodium nitroprusside, may be required. Blood pressure must be reduced slowly, because reducing it too quickly may cause hypoperfusion of organs, with the risk of cerebral infarction and blindness, deterioration of renal function, and myocardial ischaemia. Predisposing factors include a history of smoking and a history of secondary hypertension.

19a. F
19b. F
19c. T
19d. T
RNA viruses include enteroviruses (poliovirus, Coxsackievirus), rotavirus, rubella, influenza, measles, mumps, RSV (respiratory syncytial virus), rabies and HIV. *Chlamydia* is an obligate intracellular bacterium. CMV (cytomegalovirus) is a DNA, herpes-type virus.

20a. T
20b. T
20c. T
20d. T
Polycythaemia may be relative (decreased plasma volume – Gaisbock's syndrome) or absolute (increased red cell mass). Absolute polycythaemia may be primary (malignant marrow stem cell overproduction of red cells) or secondary. Causes of secondary polycythaemia include smoking, obesity, chronic lung/heart disease or any cause of raised erythropoietin production, e.g. renal carcinoma. Primary absolute polycythaemia may also be associated with increased white cell and platelet numbers, and typically presents with thrombotic symptoms, e.g. stroke, but may also present with bleeding

although this is much less common. Treatment involves removing the offending cause where possible (stop smoking, lose weight), or, for those individuals who are symptomatic, phlebotomy.

21a. F
21b. T
21c. T
21d. F
Lidocaine (lignocaine) works by blocking inactivated Na^+ channels, which are greater in number in ischaemic areas after myocardial infarction. It has a duration of action of approximately 20 minutes after intravenous injection.

22a. F
22b. T
22c. T
22d. F
Lung compliance is the change in volume per unit change in pressure. In emphysema, as a result of destruction of lung parenchyma, the lungs are easier to distend, and compliance is greater. Increased compliance is seen with advancing age. Increased interstitial fluid makes lungs 'stiffer' – decreased compliance. Decreased compliance is also associated with lung fibrosis.

23a. T
23b. T
23c. T
23d. F
The large intestine consists of the caecum, the appendix, and the ascending, transverse, descending and sigmoid colon. The psoas muscle is closely related to the caecum and appendix, so infection and perforation can result in a psoas abscess. The inferior mesenteric artery supplies the intestine from the distal third of the transverse colon to the rectum. The large intestine receives its sympathetic supply from T10–L2 and therefore refers pain to these dermatomes. McBurney's point is the site at which the base of the appendix lies. It is one-third of the way along the oblique line, joining the right anterosuperior iliac spine to the umbilicus.

24a. T
24b. F
24c. T
24d. F
β-Adrenergic receptors are of two main types: type 1 (located in the heart) and type 2 (located in the airways and peripheral vasculature). There are also β receptors in the pancreas and liver. They may be inhibitory or excitatory and act via the activation of adenylyl cyclase and a release of cAMP. Drugs used in asthma are β agonists and cause smooth muscle relaxation in the bronchi.

25a. T
25b. T
25c. F
25d. F
The five compartments of the hand are the thenar, hypothenar, central, adductor and bone. The central compartment contains the mid-palmar space and the thenar compartment contains the thenar space. Infection in the hand can easily spread to the forearm via the carpal tunnel. The fibrous lateral septum divides the central and thenar compartments and runs from the lateral border of the palmar aponeurosis to the third, not the second, metacarpal.

26a. T
26b. T
26c. F
26d. F
The adrenal gland contains a central medulla and a surrounding cortex responsible for corticosteroid production from cholesterol.

The cortex is divided into three zones, which from the outermost layer are as follows:

- The zona glomerulosa is the main site for production of mineralocorticoids: mainly aldosterone, which plays an important role in the body's Na^+ homoeostasis (regulated through the renin–angiotensin II pathway). Sodium homoeostasis is important not only for nerve function, but also for blood osmolarity and pressure.
- The zona fasciculata is responsible for producing glucocorticoids. Cortisol is the main glucocorticoid produced in humans; it influences carbohydrate metabolism. Cortisol secretion is stimulated by ACTH, from the anterior pituitary, by binding to a cell-surface receptor and in turn increasing intracellular cAMP.
- The zona reticularis acts as a small production site for androgens; dihydroepiandrosterone (DHEA) is the main secretion.

27a. T
27b. T
27c. T
27d. T
The cavernous sinuses are located on either side of the sella turcica on the upper surface of the sphenoid bone. From inferior to superior the lateral wall of the cavernous sinus incorporates the trigeminal, trochlear and oculomotor nerves. The abducens nerve, along with the internal carotid artery, also passes through the sinus. The facial vein drains into the cavernous sinus via the superior ophthalmic vein, so any infection involving the danger triangle of the face, which runs from the medial angle of the eyes along the nose to the lateral angle of the upper lip, may spread to the cavernous sinus and from there to the meninges.

28a. T
28b. F
28c. T
28d. T
The summary of antibacterial therapy in Chapter 5 of the *British National Formulary* (BNF) is required knowledge for the MCEM Part A exam. Recommended antibiotics for community-acquired pneumonia are amoxicillin or erythromycin (if penicillin allergic), or cefotaxime and erythromycin in severe cases. Quinolones such as ciprofloxacin are recommended as part of an antibiotic regimen in hospital-acquired pneumonia.

29a. F
29b. F
29c. T
29d. T
In PNH there is a clone of abnormal haematopoietic stem cells resulting in red cells with an abnormal surface, rendering them sensitive to complement. The term 'nocturnal' refers to the belief that haemolysis is triggered by acidosis during sleep and activates complement to haemolyse an unprotected and abnormal red cell membrane. However, this observation was later disproved. Haemolysis is shown to occur throughout the day and is not actually paroxysmal, but the urine concentrated overnight produces the dramatic, dark, early-morning urine. Presentation is usually with anaemia and intravascular haemolysis. There is often mild jaundice, haemoglobinuria, hepatosplenomegaly and venous thromboses in large vessels, e.g. the hepatic vein. The neutrophil alkaline phosphatase score is low and Ham's test is positive (increased sensitivity to lysis in acidified serum). (Ham's test is the definitive test of diagnosing paroxysmal nocturnal haemoglobinuria (PNH). The red cells are tested for resistance to lysis during incubation with acidified fresh serum. Lowering of pH results in complement lysis of red cells with the PNH defect.) Treatment is usually supportive but stem cell transplantation is curative in those with severe disease.

30a. T
30b. F
30c. T
30d. T
Both insulin and glucagon, together with somatostatin, are secreted from the islets of Langerhans in the pancreas. α Cells produce glucagon and sit in the periphery of the islets together with the δ cells that produce somatostatin. The central β cells produce insulin. Both insulin and glucagon are secreted as pre-hormones.

Essentially insulin is anabolic and glucagon catabolic.

The effects are summarised below.

Insulin
Stimulates synthesis of triglycerides (TGs) from free fatty acids (FFAs) and inhibits release of FFAs from TGs.

Increases synthesis of hepatic glycogen and thereby glucose uptake and storage.

Inhibits hepatic gluconeogenesis, thus saving amino acids.

Stimulates glucose uptake in skeletal muscle, which is stored as glycogen and used in energy metabolism.

Stimulates amino acid uptake in skeletal muscle and is essential for protein synthesis.

Reduces hunger by a hypothalamic effect on the brain.

Glucagon

Stimulates release of FFAs from TGs.

Stimulates glycogenolysis and glucose release.

Stimulates gluconeogenesis.

31a. T
31b. T
31c. T
31d. T

The right kidney usually lies slightly inferior to the left kidney because of the large size of the right lobe of the liver. Renal pathology may result in hip pain as a result of the close relationship of the kidneys to psoas major. Rupture of the intermediate part of the urethra results in the extravasation of urine and blood into the deep perineal pouch, which passes superiorly and extraperitoneally around the prostate and bladder. Rupture of the spongy urethra results in extravasation of urine into the superficial perineal space; the attachments of the perineal fascia determine the direction of flow of the extravasated urine.

32a. F
32b. T
32c. F
32d. T

Helicobacter pylori infects the upper GI (gastrointestinal) tract. It is a flagellated bacterium that burrows through the stomach mucus to the epithelial cells. Ammonia production, by the breakdown of urea by urease, protects *H. pylori* from the acidic environment. Most infections are asymptomatic but infection is associated with peptic ulcer disease and gastric malignancy.

33a. T
33b. T
33c. F
33d. F

Neutrophils are increased in bacterial infection, trauma, surgery, inflammation, burns, AMI, myeloproliferative disorders, steroid use and malignancy. They are decreased in viral infections, TB, drugs (carbimazole), hypersplenism, and vitamin B_{12} and folate deficiency. Lymphocytes are increased in viral infections, brucellosis, toxoplasmosis and CLL. They are decreased in steroid therapy, SLE, AIDS and post-chemotherapy treatment. Eosinophils are raised in asthma and atopic conditions but are not pathognomonic.

34a. F
34b. F
34c. F
34d. F
The following table shows how test results may be described in our fictional example:

	Ischaemic heart disease	
Procalysis	Present	Absent
Positive	200 = true positives	50 = false positives
Negative	300 = false negatives	150 = true negatives

The number of people with the disease is the true positives + false negatives = 500.

The specificity is the number of true negatives/the *total* number of negative results = 150/200 = 75%.

35a. F
35b. T
35c. T
35d. T
Many drugs may cause bradycardia, even at therapeutic levels. This may be a desired effect as part of treatment, e.g. with β blockers (e.g. sotalol) or digoxin, or part of the substance's wider actions on receptors (e.g. clonidine, opiates and alcohol). Tricyclic antidepressants such as amitriptyline cause tachycardia due to anticholinergic effects.

36a. T
36b. T
36c. F
36d. T
Diabetes insipidus results from either reduced vasopressin secretion from the pituitary (e.g. after head injury, tumour or meningitis) or a reduced response of the kidney to vasopressin (e.g. lithium therapy, hypercalcaemia, hypokalaemia and pyelonephritis). It usually presents with polyuria and polydipsia.

The serum osmolarity is usually high (low suggests psychogenic polydipsia) and that of the urine low. The water deprivation test is usually diagnostic.

37a. F
37b. T
37c. F
37d. T
Multiple myeloma is a B-cell malignancy of the plasma cells. These proliferate in the marrow, resulting in failure. There is usually a decreased albumin level and increased protein levels due to high immunoglobulins, which on electrophoresis are usually IgG. IgM is the rarest form. Light chains are precipitated in

the urine (Bence Jones proteins). Bone destruction with lytic lesions is common, resulting in hypercalcaemia, which may lead to renal failure (also caused by hyperuricaemia, UTIs and light chain precipitation). Neurological problems often occur secondary to plasmacytomas. The ESR is usually extremely high. Treatment usually is symptomatic with radiotherapy for bone pain.

38a. F
38b. T
38c. T
38d. F
Metformin is a biguanide that acts by increasing the peripheral utilisation of glucose and decreasing the absorption of glucose from the GI tract and gluconeogenesis. It does not cause hypoglycaemia. It may cause a lactic acidosis (which will give a raised anion gap). Sulphonylureas, such as glibenclamide, stimulate release of endogenous insulin from the pancreas and therefore require functioning β cells. They may also decrease breakdown of insulin and increase the density of insulin receptors on the cell.

39a. F
39b. T
39c. T
39d. F
Tetanus is infection with the Gram-positive organism *Clostridium tetani*. The site of infection is not always obvious because the spores can lie dormant for a long period. Once activated, tetanospasmin results in muscle spasm and the shorter nerves tend to be affected first; hence lockjaw, and the need for a surgical airway will be high because the patient often cannot be intubated.

High-risk groups include those never immunised, those with lapsed immunisation, e.g. elderly people, and people who are intravenous (IV) drug abusers.

Once a person is infected, life-long immunity does not occur.

40a. F
40b. T
40c. F
40d. T
Collagen is synthesised by fibroblasts. There are many types of collagen (28) but most are types I, II, III or IV. Osteogenesis imperfecta is a disease affecting collagen type I. The collagen protein is unusual in that it has the amino acid glycine at every third location. Vitamin C is a cofactor required for collagen synthesis and deficiency results in scurvy.

41a. F
41b. T
41c. F
41d. F
Femoral nerve damage results in anterior thigh sensory loss and weakness of knee extensors. Sciatic nerve injury causes posterior thigh sensory

symptoms and loss of power to muscles in the posterior thigh. The superficial peroneal nerve supplies sensation to the lateral aspect of the lower leg and dorsum of the foot. Its motor function is to evert the foot. The deep peroneal nerve supplies sensation to the first toe web space.

42a. T
42b. F
42c. T
42d. F
Sodium bicarbonate infusions generate CO_2, exacerbating intracellular acidosis. Although used in the management of hyperkalaemia, it should never be mixed with calcium-containing fluids because calcium carbonate (chalk) precipitates out. Solutions are hypernatraemic and hyperosmolar, causing marked tissue damage if extravasation occurs. Sodium bicarbonate is useful in the management of tricyclic antidepressant overdose, reducing cardiac toxicity by increasing protein binding.

43a. T
43b. F
43c. T
43d. T
Aortic dissection is associated with connective tissue diseases, Marfan's syndrome, Ehlers–Danlos syndrome, bicuspid aortic valves, smoking, crack cocaine use, hypertension and trauma.

Stroke-like presentations occur when the dissection involves the carotid arteries; paraplegia with sensory loss may result if spinal arteries are occluded. Dissections should be suspected in 'stroke patients' with pain.

44a. T
44b. T
44c. T
44d. T
The risk of bleeding in patients also taking warfarin can be increased by many mechanisms and medications. Note that the question did not ask which of the medications caused an increase in INR (international normalised ratio), but which caused an increased bleeding risk.

The risk is increased, without a concomitant elevation of the INR, by drugs that interfere with platelet aggregation (including aspirin, clopidogrel and antidepressants [particularly selective serotonin reuptake inhibitors]) and by non-steroidal anti-inflammatory drugs (NSAIDs), which can cause erosions in the gastrointestinal tract. Drugs that interfere with intestinal synthesis of vitamin K may enhance the response to warfarin; these include many antibiotics that alter the balance of the intestinal flora. Some antibiotics, such as co-trimoxazole, metronidazole, macrolides and fluoroquinolones, also inhibit the hepatic metabolism of warfarin through inhibition of the cytochrome P450 isoenzyme, which can potentiate the effects of warfarin and requires warfarin dose reduction in most cases. Paracetamol can increase the INR in patients taking warfarin, through interruption of the vitamin K cycle.

45a. T
45b. F
45c. F
45d. F
In a normal distribution the mean, mode and median are all equal. Ninety-five per cent of observations lie within 1.96 standard deviations of the mean. The Mann–Whitney test is used for non-parametric data.

46a. F
46b. T
46c. F
46d. F
The medial meniscus is attached to the medial collateral ligament but the lateral meniscus is not attached to the lateral collateral ligament. Popliteus acts when the knee is locked to rotate the femur laterally 5° on the tibial plateau, thus unlocking the knee and allowing flexion to occur. The anterior cruciate ligament (ACL) arises from the anterior intercondylar area of the tibia. It extends posteriorly, superiorly and laterally to insert into the posterior part of the medial side of the lateral condyle of the femur. The posterior cruciate ligament arises from the posterior intercondylar area of the tibia, and passes superiorly and anteriorly on the medial side of the ACL to attach to the anterior part of the lateral surface of the medial condyle of the femur. The knee has eight bursae (suprapatellar, popliteus, anserine, gastrocnemius, semimembranous, prepatellar, infrapatellar and deep infrapatellar), four of which communicate with the synovial cavity of the knee (suprapatellar, popliteus, anserine and gastrocnemius).

47a. F
47b. T
47c. F
47d. F
This patient has a respiratory acidosis probably as a result of acute or chronic pulmonary disease.

Although these patients should be given high-flow oxygen, if their PaO_2 is extremely low and as this patient is not particularly hypoxic but does have an excessively high $PaCO_2$, their oxygen should be limited to 24% or 28%. There is evidence of compensation seen in the elevated bicarbonate level. This will help reduce the CO_2 level and hopefully help to improve the conscious level.

48a. F
48b. T
48c. T
48d. F
The innate immune system comprises phagocytes (neutrophils, macrophages and monocytes, eosinophils, basophils, and dendritic and NK or natural killer cells), complement and acute phase reactants. It mounts the initial, non-specific response. Macrophages are fixed in lymphoid and mucosal tissue, whereas monocytes circulate. Within the adaptive immune response the antibody-producing B cells comprise approximately 25% of the lymphocytes.

49a. T
49b. F
49c. F
49d. T

Staphylococcus aureus is a coagulase-positive, Gram-positive coccus. Twenty-five per cent of the population are permanent carriers. *Staph. aureus* food poisoning follows ingestion of food contaminated with preformed, heat-stable enterotoxins, and symptoms appear early, approximately 1–6 hours after ingestion.

50a. F
50b. T
50c. F
50d. F

Noradrenaline (norepinephrine) acts via α_1-receptors to cause vasoconstriction. β_2-Receptor stimulation increases heart rate and contractility. β_2-Receptor stimulation dilates blood vessels in skeletal muscle and the liver. Adrenaline is the principal catecholamine secreted from the medulla, with noradrenaline and dopamine in smaller amounts.